# 101 ROMANTIC Short Stories

Short Stories for Seniors

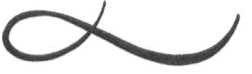

**seniorality**

101 Romantic Short Stories for Seniors -
Jamie Stonebridge, Sam Suncroft
Copyright © 2024
Seniorality / Everbreeze Media Oy

The stories presented in this book are based on factual research and historical records. While every effort has been made to ensure accuracy, the narratives contained herein are interpretations of
real events and individuals.

Set in 16 pt EB Garamond

# 1. A Million Dollar Plan

In the bustling streets of New York City, where the skyline stretched high into the clouds and the hustle and bustle of life never ceased, lived a trio of ambitious young women: Lucy, Jane, and Kate. They were determined to make a name for themselves in the big city, with dreams as vast as the skyscrapers that loomed overhead.

One day, over brunch at their favorite café, the three friends made a pact – they would marry millionaires and live a life of luxury and glamour. With their charm, wit, and beauty, they were certain they could catch the eye of a wealthy suitor and secure their futures once and for all.

Their plan was simple: they would frequent the most exclusive clubs and events, dressed to the nines and ready to dazzle any man who crossed their path. They would bat their eyelashes and flash their smiles, all the while keeping their sights set on the ultimate prize – a millionaire husband.

But as they delved deeper into their scheme, they soon realized that finding true love was not as easy as it seemed. Along the way, they encountered men who were more interested in their bank accounts than their hearts, and they began to question whether their quest for wealth was worth sacrificing their dignity and integrity.

As they navigated the treacherous waters of high society, Lucy, Jane, and Kate discovered that the most valuable treasure of all was the bond of friendship they shared. Through thick and thin, they stood by each other's side, offering support and encouragement when the going got tough.

And in the end, it wasn't a millionaire who captured their hearts, but three ordinary men who loved them for who they truly were – flaws and all. With their newfound perspective, Lucy, Jane, and Kate realized that happiness couldn't be bought with money, but earned through love, laughter, and the unbreakable bond of friendship.

# 2. A Bouquet of Secrets

In the small town of Upwood, where gossip bloomed like wildflowers in spring, lived two teenagers, Lily and Jack. Lily was a shy girl with a fondness for books, while Jack was the captain of the football team, with a heart as big as his muscles. They had been neighbors since they were kids, their houses separated by a picket fence covered in ivy.

One sunny afternoon, while Lily was tending to her garden of roses, Jack leaned over the fence, a bashful smile on his face. "Hey, Lily," he called out, his voice carrying over the gentle breeze.

Lily looked up, her cheeks turning pink. "Hi, Jack. What brings you here?"

Jack scratched the back of his neck nervously. "Well, I, uh, I wanted to ask you something."

Lily's heart skipped a beat. "Sure, what is it?"

Jack took a deep breath. "I was wondering if you'd like to go to the spring dance with me?"

Lily's eyes widened in surprise. She had always admired Jack from afar, but she never imagined he would ask her out. "I-I'd love to," she stammered, her smile brightening the garden even more.

As the days passed, the anticipation of the dance filled the air. Lily couldn't help but feel butterflies fluttering in her stomach whenever she thought about going with Jack. Meanwhile, Jack found himself daydreaming about Lily's radiant smile and the way her eyes sparkled in the sunlight.

On the night of the dance, Lily stood in front of her mirror, nervously adjusting her dress. She had chosen a simple floral dress that matched the beauty of her garden. Just as she was about to leave, there was a knock on the door.

Opening it, she found Jack standing there, holding a bouquet of daisies. "These are for you," he said, his cheeks tinged with pink.

Lily's heart melted at the sight of the flowers. "Thank you, Jack. They're beautiful."

Together, they walked to the dance, their laughter mingling with the sound of music drifting from the gymnasium. As they danced under the twinkling lights, Lily felt like she was floating on air, her worries melting away in Jack's arms.

But beneath the surface of their budding romance, secrets lurked, waiting to be revealed. Unbeknownst to Lily, Jack had been harboring a secret crush on her for years, while Lily had been too shy to admit her feelings for Jack.

As the night wore on, their feelings finally came to light, and they shared a tender kiss under the moonlit sky. In that moment, surrounded by the scent of flowers and the sound of their beating hearts, Lily and Jack knew that their love would bloom forever, just like the roses in Lily's garden.

# 3. Racing Hearts

In the heart of the American South, where the roar of engines filled the air and the smell of gasoline lingered like a promise of excitement, lived a young woman named Lisa. She was a mechanic at the local racing circuit, with grease under her fingernails and a passion for speed that matched the fastest cars on the track.

One day, as she worked tirelessly in the garage, Lisa crossed paths with Mike, a talented but reckless race car driver with a reputation for living life in the fast lane. Sparks flew between them from the moment they met, their chemistry undeniable as they bantered back and forth beneath the hood of a souped-up muscle car.

Despite their differences, Lisa and Mike found themselves drawn to each other like magnets, their shared love of racing forging a bond that was as strong as steel. Together, they worked tirelessly to prepare for the upcoming championship race, each determined to prove themselves on the track and in each other's hearts.

But their romance was tested when a rival driver, jealous of Mike's talent and success, sought to sabotage their chances of winning. As tensions mounted and danger loomed on the horizon, Lisa and Mike were forced to confront their fears and fight for their dreams – both on and off the racetrack.

In the end, it wasn't the thrill of victory or the glory of the championship that mattered most, but the love that had blossomed between them amidst the roar of engines and the scent of burning rubber. And as they sped across the finish line hand in hand, Lisa and Mike knew that their love was the greatest prize of all.

## 4. A Taste of Equality

In the bustling city of Brooksville, where the streets hummed with the rhythm of progress, lived two young souls, Emma and Michael. Emma was a fiery redhead with a passion for justice, while Michael was a dashing lawyer with a heart as vast as the courtroom. Their paths crossed one fateful day when Emma stormed into Michael's office, demanding justice for a case close to her heart.

Emma slammed a newspaper down on Michael's desk, her eyes blazing with determination. "You have to help me," she exclaimed, her voice echoing through the room.

Michael raised an eyebrow, intrigued by the fiery young woman standing before him. "What seems to be the problem?"

Emma took a deep breath, her hands trembling with anger. "My friend, Sarah, is being unfairly accused of a crime she didn't commit. She needs someone to defend her in court."

Michael studied Emma for a moment, impressed by her unwavering spirit. "I'll take the case," he declared, a hint of admiration in his voice.

As they worked together to prepare Sarah's defense, Emma and Michael found themselves drawn to each other in ways they couldn't explain. Despite their differences, they shared a common goal: to fight for justice and equality in a world that often seemed stacked against them.

As the trial unfolded, Emma and Michael stood side by side in the courtroom, their passion igniting sparks of change in the air. With Michael's legal expertise and Emma's fiery rhetoric, they fought tooth and nail to prove Sarah's innocence.

When the trial drew to a close, tensions ran high, threatening to tear Emma and Michael apart. In a moment of heated debate, they found themselves at odds, their opposing viewpoints driving a wedge between them.

It wasn't until they faced their own vulnerabilities and insecurities that they realized the true depth of their connection. In a heartfelt moment of honesty, Emma and Michael laid bare their fears and doubts, opening their hearts to each other in ways they never thought possible.

In the end, justice prevailed, and Sarah was acquitted of all charges. But more importantly, Emma and Michael discovered that they were stronger together than they ever were apart. As they walked hand in hand into the sunset, they knew that their love would always be a force to be reckoned with, just like the pursuit of equality they shared.

## 5. Sweet Home Tennessee

In the heart of the rolling hills of Tennessee, where the air was thick with the scent of magnolias and the sound of bluegrass music filled the air, lived a young woman named Mary. She was a country girl through and through, with a smile as bright as the summer sun and a spirit as free as the wind.

One day, while she was out exploring the hillsides, Mary stumbled upon a stranger – a handsome young man named Sam. He was a city boy, visiting his family's cabin for the summer, with a charm that matched his southern drawl.

Despite their different upbringings, Mary and Sam found themselves drawn to each other. They would spend hours exploring the countryside together, their laughter echoing through the hills like the call of the whippoorwill.

As the days turned into weeks, Mary found herself falling for Sam, his easygoing nature and quick wit stealing her heart. And though she tried to deny her feelings, she couldn't help but blush whenever he flashed her that crooked smile of his.

But their budding romance was threatened when Mary's family revealed a long-held secret – Sam was her distant cousin, come to Tennessee to claim his share of the family inheritance.

At first, Mary was devastated. How could she have fallen for someone who was practically family? But as she watched Sam struggle with his own feelings, she realized that their love was too strong to be denied.

Together, they faced the disapproval of their families and the gossip of the townsfolk, determined to prove that their love was worth fighting for. And as they danced beneath the stars on warm summer nights, Mary knew that she had found her home in Sam's arms.

In the end, it wasn't the blood that bound them together, but the love they shared for each other and the land that they called home. And as they stood hand in hand, watching the fireflies dance in the twilight, Mary knew that their love would endure, like the sweet sound of a fiddle playing in the Tennessee hills.

## 6. Summer Breezes

In the sun-kissed paradise of Seaview Beach, where the waves danced to the rhythm of the ocean and laughter filled the air, lived two teenagers swept up in a whirlwind of adventure: Mia and Leo. Mia was a vibrant dancer with a passion for exploration, while Leo was a carefree surfer with a heart as boundless as the sea.

Their story began on a balmy summer day, when Mia's family rented a beach house next to Leo's. With the salty breeze tousling their hair and the sand warm beneath their feet, they found themselves drawn to each other like moths to a flame, eager to explore the wonders of the seaside together.

As the days stretched into weeks, Mia and Leo's friendship blossomed into something more, their laughter mingling with the sound of crashing waves and seagulls soaring overhead. Together, they rode the waves, danced beneath the stars, and chased sunsets along the shore, their hearts brimming with the promise of endless summer days.

Amidst the carefree bliss of their seaside paradise, Mia and Leo found themselves facing obstacles that threatened to dampen their spirits. Mia's fear of the ocean, stemming from a childhood trauma, clashed with Leo's love for surfing, leading to tension that lingered beneath the surface of their idyllic romance.

Mia confided in Leo about her fear, laying bare the scars that had long haunted her. With compassion and understanding, Leo vowed to help her overcome her fear, offering his unwavering support and encouragement.

Together, Mia and Leo embarked on a journey of healing and self-discovery, their bond growing stronger with each passing day. With Leo's patient guidance and Mia's unwavering determination, they conquered her fear of the ocean, transforming it into a source of joy and freedom.

As the summer drew to a close, Mia and Leo stood hand in hand on the shore, watching the sun dip below the horizon in a blaze of fiery hues. In that moment, surrounded by the beauty of nature and the warmth of their love, they knew that their summer romance was just the beginning of a lifetime of adventures together, under the endless skies of Seaview Beach.

## 7. Love in the Fields

In the heart of rural Texas, where the land stretched far and wide under the Texan sun, there lived a young man named Luke. He was a farmer, tilling the soil day in and day out, his hands calloused from hard work, but his heart gentle and kind.

One summer, while he was out in the fields, Luke met Sarah. She was the daughter of a wealthy landowner, visiting her family's property for the season. Sarah was unlike anyone Luke had ever met – with her grace and elegance, she seemed out of place among the rows of corn and cotton.

Despite their differences in background, Luke and Sarah formed an unlikely friendship. They would meet in secret, away from the prying eyes of the townsfolk, and talk for hours about their hopes and dreams.

As the days passed, Luke found himself falling for Sarah, enchanted by her beauty and spirit. He would steal glances at her whenever he could, his heart skipping a beat whenever their eyes met.

But their love was not without its challenges. Sarah's family looked down upon Luke, considering him beneath their station. And Luke knew that he could never offer Sarah the kind of life she was accustomed to.

Yet, despite the obstacles in their path, Luke and Sarah's love only grew stronger with each passing day. They would steal moments together in the fields, their laughter ringing out like music in the warm Texas air.

But their happiness was short-lived. One fateful day, tragedy struck, tearing them apart and leaving Luke to face the harsh realities of life alone.

Years went by, and Luke never forgot Sarah – the girl who had stolen his heart amidst the fields of Texas. And though their love had been forbidden, it had left an indelible mark on his soul, shaping him into the man he had become.

Then, one day, as Luke stood in the fields, lost in memories of days gone by, he saw a figure approaching in the distance. It was Sarah, her face etched with lines of sorrow and regret.

Without a word, they ran into each other's arms, their love rekindled in an instant. And as they stood together in the fading light of day, Luke knew that their love was like a giant – unyielding and everlasting, despite the trials and tribulations they had faced.

## 8. Love's Gentle Snare

In the bustling halls of McKinley High, where laughter echoed and lockers clanked shut, there existed an unspoken tension between two souls: Sarah, with her cascading chestnut locks and eyes like dew-kissed emeralds, and Mark, the charming quarterback with a smile that could melt glaciers.

It all began on a crisp autumn afternoon, amidst the fluttering leaves and whispered secrets of the school courtyard. Sarah, lost in the melody of her favorite book, found herself bumping into Mark, who was engrossed in a football playbook.

Their eyes met, sparking a connection that neither could deny. Mark's heart quickened, and Sarah felt a warmth spreading through her like wildfire. With a bashful smile, Mark offered to walk Sarah to her next class, and she accepted, her heart fluttering like a trapped butterfly.

As they strolled side by side, their conversations flowed effortlessly, weaving dreams of the future and sharing snippets of their innermost thoughts. Mark discovered Sarah's passion for poetry, while Sarah marveled at Mark's love for astronomy. With each passing day, their bond grew stronger, like vines intertwining in a gentle embrace.

Despite their growing affection, doubts lingered in the shadows of their hearts. Mark, hesitant to confess his feelings, feared rejection, while Sarah, scarred by past heartaches, was wary of opening her heart again.

But fate had other plans.

One fateful afternoon, during a heated game against their rival school, Mark suffered a sprained ankle, leaving him sidelined and crestfallen. Sarah, witnessing his distress from the bleachers, felt a surge of empathy coursing through her veins.

Summoning her courage, Sarah approached Mark after the game, offering words of encouragement and a sympathetic ear. Mark, touched by her kindness, felt a warmth spreading through him like a comforting blanket.

In that vulnerable moment, walls crumbled, and hearts collided.

With trembling hands and bated breath, Mark poured out his feelings to Sarah, confessing his love in a torrent of emotion. Sarah, her heart overflowing with joy, reciprocated his feelings with tears glistening in her eyes.

And in that tender embrace, amidst the cheers of victory and the whispers of the wind, they found solace in each other's arms.

From that day forth, Sarah and Mark became inseparable, their love blossoming like a delicate rose in the garden of their hearts. And as they walked hand in hand, beneath the starlit sky, they knew that their love was a gift worth cherishing for eternity.

## 9. A Dream in Paris

In the romantic streets of Paris, where the Eiffel Tower stood tall against the azure sky and the Seine river flowed like a ribbon of silver, lived a young American artist named David. He had come to Paris with dreams of capturing the city's beauty on canvas, his heart brimming with hope and ambition.

One day, as he wandered the cobblestone streets of Montmartre, David crossed paths with Lise, a captivating young woman with a grace and elegance that took his breath away. She moved with the fluidity of a dancer, her laughter like music in the air, and David was instantly captivated by her charm.

Despite the language barrier and the differences in their backgrounds, David and Lise formed a connection that transcended words. They would spend hours together, wandering the streets of Paris, their hearts entwined in the magic of the city's enchanting beauty.

But their budding romance was soon overshadowed by the presence of another man – Henri, a wealthy suitor who sought Lise's hand in marriage. Though David was torn by jealousy and doubt, he knew that he couldn't stand in the way of Lise's happiness, even if it meant sacrificing his own.

As the streets of Paris became a battleground for love and desire, David and Lise found themselves caught in a whirlwind of emotion, torn between duty and passion. And as they walked beneath the starlit sky, their hearts heavy with longing, they realized that true love was worth fighting for – even in the face of seemingly insurmountable odds.

In the end, it was a chance encounter at the ballet that brought David and Lise together once more, their love stronger than ever in the glow of the stage lights. And as they embraced in the moonlit streets of Paris, surrounded by the echoes of their dreams, they knew that their love was a masterpiece – a work of art that would endure for eternity.

## 10. Second Chance at Love

In the quaint town of Woodford, Lily Evans walked along the cobbled streets, her heart aflutter with anticipation. It had been a year since her husband, James, disappeared during a fishing trip. She had searched tirelessly for him, clinging to the hope that he would return. But as time passed, the townsfolk whispered that she should move on.

One sunny afternoon, as Lily passed by the town square, she spotted a familiar face - Jack Thompson. Jack was James's best friend, and he had been a pillar of support during Lily's darkest days. They exchanged warm smiles, but beneath Jack's cheerful demeanor, Lily sensed a hint of sadness.

"Hey, Lily," Jack said, his voice tinged with longing. "How have you been holding up?"

Lily shrugged, forcing a smile. "Taking it one day at a time, Jack. How about you?"

Jack hesitated before replying, "I've been managing, but... I miss James, too."

Their shared grief brought them closer together, and soon they found solace in each other's company. They reminisced about the adventures they had shared with James, laughing through tears as they recounted his antics.

As the days passed, Lily found herself drawn to Jack in ways she hadn't expected. His kindness and understanding filled the void in her heart, and she couldn't help but wonder if love could blossom anew.

One evening, under the starlit sky, Lily and Jack sat on the porch swing, lost in conversation. The air was filled with the sweet scent of jasmine, and the gentle breeze stirred the leaves of the old oak tree.

"Lily," Jack began, his voice hesitant. "I know it's been hard for both of us, but... I've realized something."

Lily turned to him, her heart racing. "What is it, Jack?"

Jack took a deep breath, his eyes reflecting the moonlight. "I've always cared about you, Lily. More than just a friend. And I can't deny that these past few months have made me realize... I love you."

Lily's breath caught in her throat, her eyes brimming with tears. Could it be true? Could she find love again after losing James?

Without a word, Lily leaned in, pressing her lips against Jack's in a tender kiss. In that moment, all the pain and sorrow melted away, leaving only the promise of a new beginning.

As they held each other close, Lily knew that James would always hold a special place in her heart. But with Jack by her side, she felt hopeful for the future, ready to embrace the second chance at love that fate had bestowed upon them.

## 11. Beachside Serenade

Along the sun-kissed shores of a picturesque coastal town, where the scent of saltwater mingled with the laughter of beachgoers, lived a young man named Mark. He was a talented musician with dreams of making it big in the music industry, his heart as free as the seagulls that soared overhead.

One summer day, as Mark lounged on the sandy beach, strumming his guitar and watching the waves roll in, he caught sight of Cindy, a vivacious young woman with a smile that lit up the shoreline. She was unlike anyone he had ever met – carefree and spontaneous, with a love for adventure that matched his own.

Drawn to her infectious energy, Mark struck up a conversation with Cindy, their laughter mingling with the sound of the surf as they whiled away the afternoon beneath the blazing sun. And as they shared stories and dreams, Mark felt a connection with Cindy that he had never experienced before.

But their budding romance was soon tested when Mark's wealthy father arranged a food festival on the beach, hoping to find a suitable match for his son among the town's elite. Caught between his father's expectations and his own desires, Mark struggled to reconcile his love for Cindy with the pressures of his privileged upbringing.

As the food festival got underway, Mark found himself torn between two worlds – the world of wealth and privilege represented by his father, and the world of freedom and love embodied by Cindy. And as tensions mounted and emotions ran high, Mark was forced to confront his own values and priorities, unsure of where his heart truly lay.

In the end, it was a heartfelt serenade beneath the stars that brought clarity to Mark's conflicted soul. With his guitar in hand and Cindy by his side, he sang of love and freedom, his voice ringing out like a beacon of hope in the darkness.

And as they danced beneath the moonlit sky, their hearts entwined in a melody of love and longing, Mark knew that he had found his true home – not in the world of wealth and privilege, but in the arms of the woman he loved, amidst the timeless beauty of the beachside serenade.

## 12. The Scarlet Siren

In the sun-drenched waters of the Caribbean, where the salty breeze carried tales of adventure and plunder, lived a daring pirate named Peter. He was a swashbuckler with a heart of gold, his spirit untamed and free as the open sea.

Peter's life changed forever when he encountered Geraldine, a fiery and fearless woman who captivated him with her strength and determination. Together, they embarked on a quest for treasure and glory, their hearts bound by the thrill of adventure and the promise of riches.

Their journey led them across the vast expanse of the ocean, as they sailed from one exotic port to another, their ship cutting through the waves like a knife through butter.

"Prepare to board, mates!" Peter shouted to his crew as they approached a merchant vessel ripe for plunder.

Geraldine stood by his side, her sword gleaming in the sunlight. "Let's show them what we're made of, Peter!"

Their daring exploits earned them a fearsome reputation among sailors and scoundrels alike, as they plundered and pillaged their way to fortune and fame.

As they faced off against rival pirates and ruthless mercenaries, Peter and Geraldine found themselves tested in ways they never could have imagined.

"We may be outnumbered, but we'll fight to the end!" Peter declared, his voice ringing out across the deck as they prepared for battle.

Geraldine nodded, her eyes blazing with determination. "We'll show them the true meaning of courage and defiance!"

Yet, through it all, their love remained as strong as the ocean currents, unyielding and unwavering in the face of danger.

In the end, it was their love that carried them through the stormy seas and treacherous waters, their hearts united against the backdrop of a world ruled by greed and ambition.

"I love you, Geraldine," Peter whispered as they stood together on the deck of their ship, the wind whipping through their hair.

Geraldine smiled, her heart full of love and devotion. "And I love you, Peter. Together, we'll conquer the seas and beyond!"

And as they set sail into the horizon, their sails billowing in the wind, Peter and Geraldine knew that their love would drive them on to the next adventure.

# 13. Lights, Camera, Love!

In the dazzling world of Broadway, where the stage was set aglow with the sparkle of sequins and the echo of applause reverberated through the air, lived a young aspiring actress named Sarah. She had dreamt of gracing the spotlight since she was a child, her heart ablaze with the passion for the theater.

One fateful day, as Sarah auditioned for a new musical production, she caught the eye of Jack, a charismatic young director with a keen eye for talent. He was captivated by Sarah's raw talent and infectious energy, and he knew in an instant that she was destined for stardom.

As rehearsals began and the curtain rose on opening night, Sarah found herself swept up in the whirlwind of the theater world, her dreams unfolding before her eyes like a technicolor spectacle. And at the center of it all was Jack, guiding her every step of the way with a steady hand and a heart full of admiration.

But their professional relationship soon blossomed into something more, as Sarah and Jack discovered a shared passion for the stage and a deepening bond that transcended the footlights. And as they danced across the boards, their hearts entwined in the magic of the theater, they realized that their love was the greatest show of all.

Yet, their romance was tested by the relentless demands of show business, as they grappled with the pressures of fame and the sacrifices it required. And as they navigated the highs and lows of their careers, Sarah and Jack found themselves at a crossroads, torn between their love for each other and their love for the stage.

In the end, it was a tender moment backstage, amidst the chaos of a sold-out performance, that brought Sarah and Jack together once more. With a whispered confession of love and a stolen kiss in the wings, they knew that no matter what challenges lay ahead, there was no business like show business – and no love quite like theirs.

# 14. A Dance to Remember

In the bustling city of Brooksville, where the streets echoed with the sounds of jazz music, there lived a young woman named Emily. With her radiant smile and graceful moves, she captivated everyone who crossed her path. But behind her cheerful facade, Emily harbored a secret longing for something more.

One evening, as Emily twirled and swayed at the local dance hall, she caught the eye of a handsome stranger named Michael. With his dark hair and piercing blue eyes, he exuded an air of mystery that drew Emily in like a moth to a flame.

Their dance was like poetry in motion, each step bringing them closer together until they were lost in a world of their own. In that moment, Emily felt alive in a way she had never experienced before.

As the night wore on, Emily and Michael shared stories of their dreams and aspirations. Michael spoke of his passion for music and his desire to travel the world, while Emily confided her longing to break free from the confines of her small town life.

With each passing moment, their connection deepened until they were inseparable. But as the dawn approached, reality came crashing down around them.

"I have to go," Michael whispered, his voice filled with regret. "But I'll never forget this night, Emily. You've changed my life in ways I can't explain."

Emily's heart sank as she watched Michael disappear into the night, leaving her alone with her thoughts and the echoes of their dance.

As time passed, Emily couldn't shake the memory of that fateful night. She longed to see Michael again, to recapture the magic they had shared on the dance floor.

Then, one day, fate intervened in the most unexpected way. Emily's best friend, Sarah, burst into her room, breathless with excitement.

"Emily, you'll never believe who's coming to perform at the dance hall tonight," Sarah exclaimed. "It's Michael! He's back in town!"

Emily's heart leaped with joy at the news. Without a moment's hesitation, she rushed to the dance hall, her pulse quickening with each step.

As she entered the dimly lit room, Emily's eyes scanned the crowd until they landed on a familiar figure standing on stage - Michael. He looked more handsome than ever, his eyes alight with anticipation as he strummed his guitar.

With a burst of courage, Emily pushed her way through the crowd until she stood before Michael, her heart pounding in her chest.

"Michael," she whispered, her voice trembling with emotion. "I never stopped thinking about you."

Michael's eyes widened in surprise, then softened with tenderness as he took Emily's hand in his own.

"Emily," he murmured, pulling her close. "I never stopped thinking about you either. Dance with me, just like old times."

And as the music swelled around them, Emily and Michael took to the dance floor once more, their bodies moving in perfect harmony. In that moment, they knew that their love was meant to last a lifetime, a timeless melody that would echo through the ages.

## 15. Wild West Hearts

In the rugged landscapes of the American West, where the mountains rose majestically against the endless expanse of sky and the air was thick with the scent of sagebrush, lived a young cowboy named Luke. He was a free spirit, roaming the open plains with his faithful horse by his side, his heart as wild as the untamed wilderness.

One day, as Luke herded cattle on his family's ranch, he crossed paths with Maggie, a spirited young woman with a fiery temper and a fierce independence that matched his own. She was unlike anyone he had ever met – unafraid to speak her mind and unapologetic in her pursuit of adventure.

Drawn to her untamed spirit, Luke found himself captivated by Maggie's charm and vitality, their hearts beating in rhythm with the pulse of the land they both called home. And as they rode across the prairie together, their laughter echoing through the canyon walls, Luke knew that he had found a kindred spirit in Maggie.

But their budding romance was soon tested when Luke's family faced financial hardship, threatening the future of their ranch. Desperate to save his family's livelihood, Luke made a deal with a wealthy landowner, agreeing to enter a high-stakes rodeo competition in exchange for much-needed funds.

As Luke trained for the rodeo, Maggie stood by his side, offering her support and encouragement every step of the way. And as the day of the competition drew near, Luke realized that his feelings for Maggie ran deeper than he had ever imagined – she was the one he wanted by his side, no matter the outcome.

In the end, it was a thrilling ride in the rodeo arena that brought Luke and Maggie together, their love as wild and untamed as the West itself. With a triumphant whoop and a heartfelt embrace, they knew that no matter what challenges lay ahead, they would face them together – two hearts united against the backdrop of the vast and beautiful wilderness they called home.

## 16. A Wild Encounter

In the quaint town of Meadowvale, where the countryside stretched for miles, lived a reserved paleontologist named David. His days were spent buried in the dusty archives of the local museum, searching for traces of ancient creatures that roamed the earth millions of years ago.

One sunny morning, as David set out on his daily expedition, he never expected that his life would be turned upside down by a chance encounter with a free-spirited woman named Sarah. With her vivacious personality and penchant for adventure, she was like a whirlwind that swept into David's ordered existence.

Their meeting was anything but ordinary. Sarah's car broke down on the side of the road, and in her frantic search for help, she stumbled upon David, who was engrossed in studying a fossilized dinosaur bone.

"Excuse me, can you help me?" Sarah exclaimed, her voice tinged with desperation.

David looked up, his brow furrowed in confusion. "I'm sorry, I'm not a mechanic."

Sarah laughed, her eyes twinkling with mischief. "No, silly! I need a ride into town. My car decided to take an unexpected nap."

Reluctantly, David agreed to give Sarah a lift, unaware of the whirlwind of chaos that was about to enter his life.

As they drove through the winding country roads, Sarah regaled David with tales of her latest escapades, from skydiving adventures to spontaneous road trips. David couldn't help but be captivated by her infectious enthusiasm, even as he struggled to keep up with her whirlwind pace.

Their journey took an unexpected turn when Sarah's pet leopard, Tiny, leaped out of the backseat, sending David's carefully laid plans into disarray. Chaos ensued as they chased Tiny through the countryside, narrowly avoiding disaster at every turn.

But amidst the mayhem, David found himself drawn to Sarah in ways he couldn't explain. Her zest for life ignited a spark within him, awakening a sense of adventure he never knew he had.

As the sun began to set on their wild escapade, David and Sarah found themselves sitting atop a hill overlooking the picturesque meadows of Meadowvale. And in that moment, surrounded by the beauty of nature, they realized that sometimes, the wildest adventures lead to the most unexpected discoveries - including love.

## 17. Tammy's Song of Love

In the tranquil bayous of Louisiana, where the moss-draped cypress trees whispered secrets to the gentle breeze and the melody of the river flowed like a timeless lullaby, lived a young girl named Tammy. She was as sweet as the honeysuckle that bloomed along the riverbanks, her heart as pure as the water that trickled through the bayou.

One day, as Tammy wandered along the banks of the river, she stumbled upon a handsome young man named Peter, stranded in the marshes after his boat had run aground. He was a wealthy landowner from the city, with a world-weary demeanor that belied a kind heart.

Drawn to Tammy's innocence and kindness, Peter found himself captivated by her gentle spirit and the simple joys of life in the bayou. Despite their differences in background and upbringing, they formed an unlikely friendship as they explored the hidden treasures of the Louisiana wilderness together.

But their bond was tested when Peter's fiancée, a glamorous socialite from the city, arrived on the scene, determined to claim him as her own. As Tammy watched from the sidelines, her heart ached with longing, knowing that she could never compete with the sophistication and wealth of Peter's world.

Yet, as the days passed and the tension between them mounted, Peter began to realize that true love was not measured in material possessions or social status, but in the depth of a person's heart. And as he looked into Tammy's eyes, he knew that he had found a love worth fighting for – a love as pure and enduring as the waters of the bayou.

In the end, it was a heartfelt confession beneath the stars that brought Peter and Tammy together, their hearts united in a song of love that echoed through the bayou. With tears of joy and laughter in their eyes, they embraced in the moonlight, knowing that they had found their happily ever after in each other's arms – a love as timeless as the river itself.

## 18. The Rebel's Resolve

In the dusty town of Dustwood, where the sun beat down mercilessly on the rugged landscape, lived a young outlaw named Jesse. With his piercing gaze and quick draw, he was known throughout the territory as the "Left-Handed Gun," a name earned for his deadly accuracy with his revolver.

Jesse's life was a series of daring escapades and narrow escapes, as he rode from town to town, always staying one step ahead of the law. But beneath his tough exterior lay a heart yearning for something more - a sense of purpose that had eluded him for too long.

One fateful day, Jesse rode into Dustwood, his eyes set on a new target - the corrupt sheriff who ruled the town with an iron fist. Determined to bring justice to the oppressed townsfolk, Jesse embarked on a mission to rid Dustwood of its tyrannical ruler once and for all.

But as Jesse plotted his next move, he found himself drawn to a fiery young woman named Alice, whose spirit matched his own in its defiance of authority. With her unruly curls and steely gaze, Alice was a force to be reckoned with, and Jesse couldn't help but admire her courage in the face of adversity.

Together, Jesse and Alice formed an unlikely alliance, their bond forged through shared hardship and a shared desire for freedom. As they plotted their rebellion against the sheriff, they grew closer with each passing day, their hearts intertwining like the tendrils of a wild vine.

But their quest for justice came at a price, as they faced danger at every turn and betrayal from unexpected quarters. And when the final showdown with the sheriff arrived, Jesse knew that he would have to confront his own demons if he ever hoped to find redemption.

With guns blazing and hearts pounding, Jesse and Alice fought side by side, their resolve unyielding in the face of adversity. And as the dust settled on the streets of Dustwood, they emerged victorious, their love a beacon of hope in a world shrouded in darkness.

In the end, Jesse realized that true strength lay not in the barrel of a gun, but in the courage to stand up for what is right, even when the odds are stacked against you. And with Alice by his side, he knew that he had finally found the purpose he had been searching for - to fight for justice, and to love without fear.

# 19. Love's Italian Symphony

In the sun-kissed city of Napoli, where the aroma of freshly baked pizza wafted through the narrow streets, lived a fiery young woman named Sophia. With her dark curls and smoldering gaze, she captured the hearts of all who crossed her path, including the wealthy businessman, Antonio.

Antonio was a man of means, his pockets lined with gold and his heart as cold as marble. But beneath his stoic exterior lay a longing for something more - a love that would set his soul on fire and fill the void in his life.

Their paths collided one fateful day when Antonio stumbled upon Sophia, singing in the piazza with a voice that stirred something deep within him. Enchanted by her beauty and captivated by her spirit, Antonio knew that he had to make her his own.

Sophia was no ordinary woman - she was a force of nature, with a fierce independence that defied tradition and convention. And as Antonio courted her with lavish gifts and declarations of love, Sophia remained resolute in her determination to chart her own destiny.

Undeterred by Sophia's resistance, Antonio devised a plan to win her heart once and for all. He proposed a marriage of convenience, a union that would secure his status in society and grant Sophia the financial security she had always dreamed of.

Beneath the veneer of their arranged marriage lay a whirlwind of passion and desire, as Sophia and Antonio navigated the highs and lows of love's Italian symphony. From heated arguments to tender moments of reconciliation, their relationship blossomed into a tempestuous affair that defied all expectations.

As the years passed, Sophia and Antonio weathered life's storms together, their love growing stronger with each passing day. And amidst the chaos of Napoli's bustling streets and the whispers of gossiping tongues, they found solace in the arms of each other, their bond unbreakable in the face of adversity.

In the end, Sophia and Antonio proved that true love knows no bounds - not wealth, not social status, not even the passage of time. For in the heart of Napoli, where passion burned brighter than the Mediterranean sun, they discovered that love was the greatest gift of all, a treasure worth fighting for until the end of time.

## 20. Paths to Prestige

In the heart of Philadelphia, where old money mingled with new aspirations, Alex sat in the bustling law firm of Preston & Sons, his brow furrowed in concentration as he pored over legal documents.

His colleague, John, leaned over from the neighboring cubicle. "Hey, Alex, heard you're heading to the St. James Gala tonight. Big night for you?"

Alex glanced up, a faint smile playing on his lips. "Yeah, Kate invited me. Should be interesting."

Later that evening, amidst the grandeur of the St. James Gala, Alex found himself amidst a sea of finely dressed socialites. Spotting Kate across the room, he made his way through the crowd.

"Alex!" Kate's voice rang out, her eyes alight with excitement as she approached him. "I'm so glad you could make it."

"Wouldn't miss it for the world," Alex replied, taking her hand in his.

As they danced to the soft strains of the orchestra, Kate leaned in close, her voice barely above a whisper. "You know, Alex, you don't have to prove anything to anyone. You're already everything I've ever wanted."

Alex's heart swelled with emotion, his doubts fading away in the warmth of Kate's embrace. "I'm just trying to find my place in this world, Kate. Sometimes it feels like I'm swimming against the current."

Kate's eyes softened with understanding. "You don't have to do it alone, Alex. We'll find our way together."

And in that moment, amidst the opulence of Philadelphia's elite, Alex realized that true success wasn't measured in wealth or status, but in the love and acceptance he found in Kate's arms. And as they continued to dance, their laughter mingling with the music, Alex knew that he had finally found his path to prestige - one that led straight to the heart of the woman he loved.

## 21. A Tale of Two Worlds

In the vibrant city of New York, where the hustle and bustle of urban life never ceased, lived two individuals from contrasting worlds - Samantha, a fiercely independent journalist, and James, a charming and suave sports columnist. Their paths collided one day at the bustling newsroom of the Daily Gazette, sparking a whirlwind romance that would challenge their perceptions of love and success.

Samantha was a force to be reckoned with, blazing trails in a male-dominated industry with her sharp wit and unwavering determination. As the "Woman of the Year" in journalism circles, she commanded respect and admiration from colleagues and readers alike. But beneath her confident facade lay a vulnerability that she kept hidden from the world, a fear of letting down her guard and allowing herself to love.

James, on the other hand, was a rising star in the world of sports journalism, effortlessly charming his way into the hearts of fans and admirers with his charismatic smile and easygoing demeanor. He thrived in the spotlight, relishing the attention and adulation that came with his success. But beneath his polished exterior lay a yearning for something more meaningful - a connection that transcended the superficialities of fame and fortune.

Their relationship was a whirlwind of passion and intensity, as Samantha and James navigated the highs and lows of love in the spotlight. From glamorous red carpet events to intimate dinners at cozy bistros, they embraced each moment with a fervor that bordered on obsession.

But as their careers soared to new heights, cracks began to form in their seemingly perfect romance. Samantha's relentless pursuit of success drove a wedge between them, while James struggled to reconcile his own ambitions with the demands of their relationship.

Amidst the chaos of their conflicting priorities, Samantha and James were forced to confront the harsh realities of love and sacrifice. And as they grappled with the choices that lay before them, they discovered that true happiness could only be found in each other's arms, where love transcended the boundaries of fame and fortune.

In the end, Samantha and James realized that their differences were what made their love so special - a union of two souls from contrasting worlds, bound together by a love that defied all expectations. And as they walked hand in hand into the sunset of their shared future, they knew that they were destined to be each other's "Person of the Year," forever and always.

## 22. Echoes of Affection

In the vibrant city of Memphis, where the rhythm of music pulsed through the streets, Johnny stepped into the dimly lit diner, his guitar slung over his shoulder. His eyes fell upon Susan, who was wiping down the counter with a gentle smile on her lips.

"Hey there, Susan," Johnny greeted, his voice warm with familiarity.

Susan glanced up, her cheeks flushing at the sight of him. "Well, if it isn't the heartthrob himself. What can I get for you today?"

"The usual, please," Johnny replied, taking a seat at the counter.

As Susan prepared his order, Johnny couldn't help but admire her grace and poise. "You know, Susan, I've been thinking about that song we were working on. I'd love to get your input on the lyrics."

Susan's eyes lit up with excitement. "Really? I'd love to help! Let's hear what you've got so far."

With a twinkle in his eye, Johnny strummed a few chords on his guitar, his voice filling the air with the soulful melody of their song. As he sang, Susan listened intently, her heart swelling with emotion at the beauty of his words.

"That was incredible, Johnny," Susan exclaimed, her eyes shining with admiration. "I can't wait to see where this song takes you, I mean us?"

Johnny smiled, his heart skipping a beat at the sound of her praise. "Thanks, Susan. I couldn't do it without you."

As they shared a moment of quiet understanding, Johnny realized that the connection he felt with Susan went beyond music - it was a bond that transcended words, a love that was as timeless as the melodies they created together.

In that dimly lit diner, amidst the hustle and bustle of the city, Johnny and Susan found solace in each other's company, their hearts beating in perfect harmony. And as they embarked on their journey together, they knew that their love would endure, a beautiful melody that would echo through the ages.

## 23. Pursuit Across Horizons

In the sprawling city of New York, where skyscrapers pierced the sky like monoliths of steel, lived an advertising executive named Roger Thornhill. With his tailored suits and quick wit, he navigated the cutthroat world of Madison Avenue with ease, his name synonymous with success and sophistication.

But Roger's life took a sudden turn when he found himself mistaken for a government agent and thrust into a world of espionage and intrigue. Pursued by enemy agents and framed for a crime he didn't commit, Roger embarked on a thrilling journey across the country, from the bustling streets of Manhattan to the vast expanse of the American heartland.

Along the way, Roger encountered a mysterious woman named Eve Kendall, whose beauty and charm captivated him from the moment they met. Despite her enigmatic nature and the secrets she held close to her chest, Roger couldn't help but be drawn to her, his heart torn between desire and suspicion.

As they raced against time to uncover the truth, Roger and Eve found themselves embroiled in a deadly game of cat and mouse, where the stakes were higher than they could have ever imagined. From the dizzying sights of Niagara Falls to the desolate beauty of the American Midwest, they traversed landscapes both breathtaking and treacherous, their bond growing stronger with each passing mile.

As they neared the truth behind the conspiracy that had engulfed them, Roger and Eve realized that they were not alone in their quest. With danger lurking around every corner and enemies closing in from all sides, they knew that they would have to rely on each other if they were to survive.

In the end, amidst the swirling chaos of their journey, Roger and Eve discovered that love could blossom in the most unexpected of places. And as they stood together, hand in hand, on the precipice of uncertainty, they knew that their bond would endure, a beacon of hope in a world shrouded in shadows.

## 24. Neon Nights and Heartfelt Risks

In the electric city of Las Vegas, where the neon lights illuminated the desert sky, lived a talented race car driver named Danny. With his fearless spirit and a need for speed, he ruled the streets and the racetracks alike, his name whispered in awe by adrenaline junkies and racing enthusiasts.

But beneath Danny's tough exterior lay a dream - to win the prestigious Las Vegas Grand Prix and prove himself as the best in the business. And when he met Scarlet, a spirited young woman with a passion for dance and a heart as vibrant as the city itself, he knew that he had found his partner in both love and competition.

Scarlet was a showgirl at the glamorous Flamingo Hotel, her dazzling smile and infectious energy lighting up the stage night after night. But beneath the glitz and glamour of her life in the spotlight, she harbored her own dreams - to dance her way to stardom and leave her mark on the world.

As Danny and Scarlet joined forces to prepare for the Grand Prix, they discovered that they shared more than just a love for speed and excitement - they shared a deep connection that transcended the boundaries of their respective worlds. From the smoky casinos to the bustling streets of the Strip, they embraced the chaos and unpredictability of Las Vegas, their passion for life fueling their drive to succeed.

But as the race drew nearer, Danny and Scarlet found themselves facing obstacles both on and off the track. From rival drivers determined to see them fail to the pressures of fame and fortune, they struggled to stay true to themselves and their dreams.

In the end, amidst the glittering lights of Las Vegas, Danny and Scarlet realized that the true prize wasn't the trophy or the accolades - it was the love they shared and the journey they had embarked upon together. And as they crossed the finish line hand in hand, they knew that their love would endure, a shining beacon of hope in a city built on dreams and desires.

## 25. Whispers of the Tropics

In the vibrant island of Trinidad, where the rhythm of steel drums filled the air, lived a woman named Mary. With her flowing dresses and infectious laughter, she captured the hearts of everyone she met, her presence like a ray of sunshine on even the cloudiest of days.

One breezy afternoon, Mary found herself at the local market, admiring the colorful array of fruits and spices. As she reached for a ripe mango, a voice behind her startled her.

"Careful there, don't want to bruise the fruit," said a deep, velvety voice.

Mary turned to see Jack, a stranger with an enigmatic smile and dark, mysterious eyes.

"Thank you," Mary replied, a hint of curiosity in her voice. "Are you from around here?"

Jack shook his head. "No, just passing through. I'm Jack."

"Mary," she introduced herself, offering a warm smile.

From that moment on, Mary and Jack found themselves drawn to each other like magnets, their conversations flowing as easily as the Caribbean breeze.

As they wandered through the bustling streets of Trinidad, Jack couldn't help but admire Mary's zest for life.

"You have a way of lighting up the room, Mary," Jack remarked, his eyes twinkling with admiration.

Mary blushed, feeling a warmth spread through her chest. "Thank you, Jack. You're not so bad yourself."

As the days turned into nights, Mary and Jack's bond deepened, their shared laughter and stolen glances speaking volumes.

One evening, as they watched the sun dip below the horizon from the edge of a secluded beach, Jack turned to Mary, his heart pounding in his chest.

"Mary, there's something I need to tell you," Jack began, his voice filled with emotion.

Mary turned to him, her eyes searching his face for answers.

"I've been keeping a secret from you," Jack confessed, his gaze never wavering from hers. "But I want you to know that it doesn't change how I feel about you."

Mary's heart skipped a beat, her mind racing with questions. "What is it, Jack? You can tell me anything."

Jack took a deep breath, his eyes shimmering in the moonlight. "I'm not who you think I am. My past is... complicated."

Mary reached out and took Jack's hand in hers, a sense of understanding washing over her. "We all have our secrets, Jack. What matters is the person you are now."

And as they watched the stars twinkle overhead, Mary and Jack knew that their love was stronger than any secret or obstacle they might face. In the embrace of the tropical night, they found solace in each other's arms, their whispers carrying on the Caribbean breeze for eternity.

# 26. Secrets Beneath the Parisian Sky

In the enchanting city of Paris, where the Eiffel Tower stood tall against the skyline, lived a woman named Claire. With her elegant grace and magnetic charm, she moved through the cobblestone streets with an air of mystery that captivated all who crossed her path.

Claire had fled to Paris to escape the ghosts of her past, seeking refuge in the beauty and romance of the City of Light. But when she met Mark, a handsome and charismatic stranger with a twinkle in his eye, her carefully constructed world was turned upside down.

Mark had a knack for charming his way into Claire's heart, his witty banter and disarming smile melting her defenses with each passing day. As they explored the charming cafes and hidden alleyways of Paris together, Claire found herself falling for him against her better judgment.

But beneath Mark's charming exterior lay a web of secrets and lies, threatening to unravel the fragile bond they had formed. From his mysterious past to the danger that lurked in the shadows, Claire realized that she didn't know Mark as well as she thought she did.

As they moved through the moonlit streets of Paris, Claire couldn't shake the feeling that something wasn't quite right. And when she stumbled upon a clue that revealed the truth about Mark's identity, she knew that she had stumbled into a dangerous game of cat and mouse.

With danger lurking around every corner and their lives hanging in the balance, Claire and Mark found themselves embroiled in a thrilling adventure that would test the limits of their courage and their love. From the rooftops of Montmartre to the opulent halls of the Louvre, they raced against time to uncover the truth and stay one step ahead of their enemies.

In the end, amidst the twinkling lights of Paris and the echoes of their shared laughter, Claire and Mark discovered that love had a way of conquering even the darkest of secrets. And as they watched the sunrise over the Seine, they knew that their bond was stronger than any obstacle they might face, a beacon of hope in a world filled with uncertainty.

# 27. A Midsummer Affair

In the quaint village of Meadowbrook, where the sun painted the fields with warm hues and the fragrance of blossoms lingered in the air, dwelled two young souls named Sophie and Ben. They were as different as chalk and cheese, yet destiny had intertwined their lives on a scorching summer's day.

Sophie was a daydreamer, often lost in the pages of novels, while Ben was a rugged lad, his hands weathered from toiling in the fields. Despite their differences, they found themselves inexplicably drawn to each other like two magnets pulled by an invisible force.

Their story unfolded one sweltering August afternoon when Sophie's bicycle broke down on the dusty road leading out of town. With no one around to assist, she felt a wave of despair until Ben appeared, his sturdy frame shining with sweat under the blazing sun.

With a bashful smile, Ben swiftly fixed her bicycle, their eyes meeting in fleeting glances as they exchanged awkward pleasantries. From that moment on, their chance encounter evolved into a friendship that flourished like the wildflowers in the meadow.

As the days stretched long under the relentless sun, Sophie and Ben sought refuge in each other's company. They explored the hidden nooks of Meadowbrook, shared secrets beneath the starry sky, and waltzed barefoot in the moonlight, their laughter mingling with the whisper of the breeze.

However, their idyllic summer was not without its challenges. Sophie's parents disapproved of her spending time with a farm boy, fearing it would distract her from her studies. Ben, too, faced pressure from his father to focus on the family farm, leaving scant time for frivolities.

Despite the obstacles, their bond only deepened with each passing day. They stole moments beneath the shade of the ancient oak tree, whispering promises of forever amidst the gentle rustle of leaves. And as the final days of summer approached, they vowed to savor every moment, aware that their time together was ephemeral.

On the eve of Sophie's departure for college, with tears glistening in her eyes and a heavy heart, she met Ben one last time by the riverbank where they had shared their first kiss. Under the waning light of the setting sun, they embraced, their love transcending time and distance.

As the seasons shifted and life led them down disparate paths, Sophie and Ben clung to the memories of that enchanted summer, knowing that regardless of where their journeys may take them, they would forever carry a piece of each other in their hearts. For in the tapestry of their lives, woven with threads of love and longing, their summer romance would forever be an indelible chapter.

## 28. A Rancher's Dilemma

In the vast expanse of the Texas plains, where the sky stretched endlessly and the wind whispered through the prairie grass, lived a rugged cowboy named Jake. He was as tough as the land he worked, yet beneath his stoic exterior lay a heart torn between duty and desire.

Jake worked tirelessly on his family's ranch, tending to the cattle and braving the elements with a resilience forged by years of hard labor. But his father, a stern man named Hank, harbored a deep distrust of modernity, clinging stubbornly to the old ways of ranching.

Their relationship was strained, marred by years of unspoken resentment and simmering tension. Jake longed to break free from his father's shadow, to carve out his own path in life, but the weight of familial expectation kept him tethered to the land he called home.

Amidst the dust and solitude of the ranch, Jake found solace in the company of Alma, a fiery young woman who worked at the local diner. She was a breath of fresh air in his world of leather and lassos, her laughter like music to his ears.

Their bond grew stronger with each stolen moment, their hearts entwined like the branches of a mesquite tree. But Alma harbored dreams of her own, dreams that beckoned her to leave behind the small town life and seek adventure in the big city.

As tensions simmered on the ranch and the specter of change loomed on the horizon, Jake found himself torn between loyalty to his family and the yearning of his heart. The arrival of Hud, Jake's reckless and charismatic younger brother, only served to exacerbate the rift between father and son.

Caught in the crossfire of their family's turmoil, Jake struggled to find his place in a world where tradition clashed with progress. But when tragedy struck the ranch, forcing Jake to confront the harsh realities of life on the frontier, he realized that sometimes, the true measure of a man lies not in the strength of his fists, but in the depth of his compassion.

In the end, Jake made a choice that defied expectations and shattered the chains of the past. With Alma by his side, he rode off into the sunset, leaving behind the dusty trails of the ranch for a future filled with hope and possibility.

As they galloped towards the horizon, their hearts soared with the promise of new beginnings, their love a beacon of light in a world shrouded in darkness. For in the vast expanse of the Texas plains, amidst the howl of the wind and the cry of the coyote, Jake and Alma found their own piece of heaven on earth.

## 29. A Stitch in Time

In the bustling streets of New York City, where the hustle and bustle of urban life never ceased, lived a talented fashion designer named Grace. She was as chic as the garments she created, her fingers nimble with needle and thread, yet beneath her polished exterior lay a heart yearning for love.

Grace lived for her art, pouring her passion into every sketch and seam, but her world was turned upside down when she crossed paths with Mike, a rough-and-tumble sportswriter with a penchant for mischief. They were as different as night and day, yet fate had a way of bringing opposites together.

Their whirlwind romance began with a chance encounter at a trendy café, where Grace's sketches caught Mike's eye as he sipped his espresso.

"Wow, these designs are incredible," Mike remarked, peering over Grace's shoulder at her sketchbook.

Grace looked up, startled by the sudden intrusion. "Oh, um, thank you," she replied, a blush creeping into her cheeks.

"Incredible doesn't even begin to describe it. You've got real talent," Mike continued, flashing her a charming grin.

Despite their clashing personalities and conflicting schedules, Grace and Mike embarked on a journey of love and laughter.

"I can't believe you've never been to a baseball game before," Mike exclaimed, his eyes lighting up with excitement.

Grace laughed, her voice tinkling like wind chimes. "Well, I've always been more of a fashion show kind of girl, but I'm willing to give it a shot."

As they navigated the highs and lows of their relationship, they soon discovered that blending their contrasting worlds was no easy feat.

"I just don't understand why you can't be more supportive of my career," Grace said, her voice tinged with frustration.

"I am supportive, Grace, but you have to understand that my job is important too," Mike replied, his brow furrowed with concern.

But through it all, they remained steadfast in their love, determined to overcome any obstacle that stood in their way.

"I know we come from different worlds, but when I'm with you, none of that seems to matter," Mike whispered, his eyes locked on Grace's.

With Grace's glamorous social circle and Mike's rough-and-tumble friends, tensions simmered beneath the surface, threatening to tear them apart.

"You don't belong with someone like him, Grace. You belong with someone who understands your world," Grace's friend remarked, her voice dripping with disapproval.

"But I love him, and that's all that matters," Grace replied, her voice filled with conviction.

In the end, Grace and Mike emerged stronger than ever, their love a testament to the power of acceptance and understanding.

"I never thought I'd find someone who gets me the way you do," Mike said, his hand intertwined with Grace's as they watched the sun set over the city skyline.

"Me neither, but I'm sure glad I did," Grace replied, her heart overflowing with happiness.

As they embraced beneath the twinkling lights of the city skyline, they knew that their love story was just beginning, with each new chapter more beautiful than the last.

# 30. September Serenade

In the picturesque countryside of Tuscany, where vineyards stretched as far as the eye could see and the aroma of ripening grapes filled the air, lived a wealthy businessman named David. He was as suave as the Italian wine he exported, his charm captivating all who crossed his path, yet beneath his sophisticated facade lay a heart yearning for something more.

David spent his summers at his lavish villa, escaping the hustle and bustle of city life in pursuit of tranquility and solitude. But his world was turned upside down when he returned one September to find unexpected guests had taken up residence in his villa.

Among them was a vibrant young woman named Sophia, whose laughter echoed through the halls and brought life to the once-empty rooms. She was as free-spirited as the breeze that danced through the olive groves, her presence stirring something deep within David's soul.

Their unexpected reunion sparked a whirlwind romance, their days filled with leisurely strolls through the vineyards and candlelit dinners under the stars.

"I never expected to find you here, Sophia," David remarked, his voice tinged with surprise as he watched her twirl beneath the moonlight.

"And I never expected to find you," Sophia replied, her eyes sparkling with mischief as she took his hand in hers.

As they explored the beauty of Tuscany together, David and Sophia discovered a connection that transcended time and space, their hearts entwined like the vines that adorned the villa's walls.

But their idyllic romance was threatened by the arrival of Maurice, Sophia's charming but persistent suitor from America.

"You can't seriously be considering going back to him, Sophia," David pleaded, his heart heavy with uncertainty.

"I don't know what to do, David. He's offering me a life of comfort and security, but my heart belongs here with you," Sophia confessed, her voice wavering with emotion.

Amidst the backdrop of the Tuscan countryside, David and Sophia grappled with their feelings, torn between the allure of the past and the promise of the future.

In the end, they chose love over convention, embracing each other beneath the Tuscan sun as they vowed to cherish every moment together.

"Our love may have started in September, but it will last a lifetime," David whispered, his arms wrapped around Sophia as they watched the sun set over the rolling hills.

And as they danced beneath the stars, their hearts beat as one, their love a testament to the power of passion and perseverance. For in the heart of Tuscany, amidst the vines and the olive trees, David and Sophia found their own slice of paradise, where love knew no bounds and every day felt like September.

# 31. Voyage of the Heart

In the bustling city of Boston, where the rhythm of life moved at a brisk pace and the harbor echoed with the calls of seagulls, lived a shy and reserved woman named Eleanor. She was as delicate as a rose in bloom, her spirit longing to break free from the confines of her sheltered existence.

Eleanor's life revolved around caring for her domineering mother, whose disapproval weighed heavy on her daughter's shoulders like a burden too great to bear. But beneath Eleanor's demure exterior lay a yearning for adventure, a longing to spread her wings and soar into the unknown.

Her chance for liberation came when she embarked on a sea voyage to South America, seeking solace and self-discovery amidst the vast expanse of the ocean.

On board the ship, Eleanor found herself drawn to a charismatic and enigmatic man named James, whose charm and wit captivated her from the moment they met.

"I must say, Miss Eleanor, you have a way with words that is quite captivating," James remarked, his eyes sparkling with intrigue as they conversed on the deck under the moonlit sky.

Eleanor blushed at his compliment, her heart fluttering like a butterfly caught in a summer breeze. "Thank you, James. It's rare to find someone who appreciates my love for literature," she replied, her voice tinged with bashfulness.

As their voyage continued, Eleanor and James forged a deep and meaningful connection, their hearts entwined like the tendrils of a vine reaching towards the sun.

But their burgeoning romance was threatened by the specter of James' troubled past and Eleanor's lingering insecurities.

"I fear that my past will always haunt me, Eleanor. I'm not sure I can ever truly escape it," James confessed, his voice heavy with regret.

"And I fear that I will never be free from the shadows of my mother's disapproval," Eleanor admitted, her eyes brimming with tears.

Amidst the ebb and flow of the ocean waves, Eleanor and James grappled with their fears and doubts, seeking solace in each other's embrace.

In the end, they chose to embrace the uncertainty of their future, setting sail towards a new horizon hand in hand, their hearts united in love and determination.

"Forget the past, Eleanor. Our journey together is just beginning," James whispered, his words carrying across the sea breeze as they watched the sun set on the horizon.

And as they sailed into the unknown, their spirits soared with the promise of new beginnings, their love a beacon of hope amidst the vastness of the ocean. For in the voyage of their hearts, Eleanor and James found the courage to chart a course towards happiness and fulfillment, leaving behind the shadows of the past to embrace the light of a brighter tomorrow.

# 32. A Season of Serendipity

In the bustling streets of New York City, where the skyline reached towards the heavens and the sounds of the city never ceased, lived a free-spirited young woman named Alice. She was as adventurous as the wind that danced through the skyscrapers, her heart yearning for excitement and spontaneity.

Alice's days were filled with societal obligations and societal expectations, but her spirit longed for something more. She dreamed of breaking free from the constraints of convention and embracing life on her own terms.

Her opportunity for liberation came when she met a charming and unconventional man named Thomas, whose zest for life and disregard for societal norms captivated her from the moment they crossed paths.

"Tell me, Alice, what is it that you truly desire in life?" Thomas asked, his eyes alight with curiosity as they strolled through Central Park.

"I want to experience everything life has to offer, to live in the moment and follow my heart wherever it may lead," Alice replied, her voice tinged with excitement.

As their whirlwind romance blossomed amidst the hustle and bustle of the city, Alice and Thomas embarked on a series of adventures, their days filled with laughter and love.

But their happiness was threatened by the expectations of Alice's wealthy and conservative family, who viewed Thomas as an unsuitable match for their daughter.

"You can't seriously be considering marrying that man, Alice. He's not of our social standing," Alice's father admonished, his voice stern with disapproval.

"But father, Thomas makes me happier than I've ever been. Can't you see that?" Alice pleaded, her heart torn between love and duty.

Amidst the pressures of society and the demands of her family, Alice grappled with the decision of whether to follow her heart or conform to the expectations placed upon her.

In the end, she chose love over convention, embracing a future with Thomas filled with passion and possibility.

"Forget what they say, Alice. Let's make our own rules and create our own happiness," Thomas whispered, his words carrying across the city streets as they danced beneath the twinkling lights of Times Square.

And as they embarked on a new chapter of their lives together, Alice and Thomas discovered that true happiness lies not in conforming to societal expectations, but in embracing the serendipity of life's unexpected twists and turns. For in their holiday of love, they found the courage to defy convention and forge their own path towards a future filled with joy and fulfillment.

## 33. Melodies of Paris

In the vibrant city of Paris, where the Seine flowed like a ribbon of silver and the streets were alive with the melodies of jazz, lived two expatriates whose souls were intertwined with the rhythm of the city.

Nina was a sultry jazz singer, her voice a mesmerizing blend of passion and melancholy, while Paul was a talented saxophonist whose melodies stirred the hearts of all who heard them. Despite their different backgrounds and the scars of their past, they found solace and inspiration in the music that bound them together.

Their romance unfolded against the backdrop of smoky jazz clubs and moonlit walks along the riverbanks, their love affair as intoxicating as the wine that flowed freely in the city of lights.

"Nina, you sing like an angel," Paul whispered, his eyes fixed on her as she performed on stage, her voice filling the room with raw emotion.

"And you play the saxophone like no one else I've ever heard," Nina replied, her heart fluttering with admiration.

But their idyllic romance was haunted by the ghosts of their pasts, as they grappled with the scars of war and the challenges of being black Americans in a city still grappling with its own prejudices.

"I can't escape the memories, Nina. The war changed me in ways I can't even begin to explain," Paul confessed, his voice tinged with pain.

"I know, Paul. But we have each other now, and together we can face anything," Nina replied, her voice filled with conviction.

As they navigated the complexities of their relationship, Nina and Paul found strength in each other's arms, their love a beacon of hope in a world filled with uncertainty.

But when an unexpected opportunity arose for Paul to return to America and pursue his dreams of fame and fortune, they were forced to confront the harsh realities of their situation.

"I can't ask you to give up your dreams for me, Paul. You have to go," Nina said, tears glistening in her eyes as she faced the prospect of losing him.

"But my dream is to be with you, Nina. Without you, none of it matters," Paul replied, his heart breaking at the thought of leaving her behind.

In the end, they chose love over ambition, embracing a future together filled with music and passion.

"Let's make beautiful music together, Nina. Wherever we go, whatever we do, as long as we're together, we'll be alright," Paul whispered, his words carrying across the Parisian night as they embraced beneath the Eiffel Tower.

And as they danced to the melodies of Paris, Nina and Paul knew that their love was a symphony worth cherishing, a testament to the power of music to heal wounds and unite souls. For in the city of love, amidst the echoes of jazz and the whispers of the wind, they found a love that would endure the test of time.

# 34. Chasing Shadows

In the sun-kissed paradise of the French Riviera, where the azure waters shimmered like liquid sapphire and the scent of Mediterranean blooms filled the air, lived a retired jewel thief named Alex. He was a man of mystery, his past shrouded in secrecy and his present a delicate balance between temptation and redemption.

Alex's tranquil existence was shattered when a series of daring heists rocked the glamorous coastal towns, leaving the authorities baffled and the local elite in a state of panic. Despite his efforts to leave his criminal past behind, Alex found himself thrust back into the dangerous world of cat and mouse, as he became the prime suspect in the robberies.

Determined to clear his name and prove his innocence, Alex embarked on a perilous quest to uncover the truth behind the crimes, enlisting the help of a spirited and enigmatic young woman named Sophie. Together, they chased shadows across the sun-drenched landscape, their hearts racing with adrenaline and their resolve tested by the allure of forbidden desires.

As they delved deeper into the mystery, Alex and Sophie found themselves drawn to each other in ways they could not explain, their partnership evolving into something more than mere allies in pursuit of justice. But as the stakes grew higher and the danger loomed ever closer, they were forced to confront their feelings and the possibility of a future together amidst the chaos and uncertainty.

In the end, Alex's quest for redemption would lead him down a path of self-discovery and transformation, as he confronted the demons of his past and embraced the promise of a new beginning. And as he stood on the cliffs overlooking the sparkling waters of the Riviera, with Sophie by his side and the sun setting in a blaze of fiery hues, he knew that their love was a beacon of hope amidst the shadows of doubt and uncertainty.

## 35. Love's Verdict

In the quaint town of Riverdale, where whispers of love floated like the delicate petals of cherry blossoms in spring, lived two souls destined to intertwine – Emily and Thomas.

Emily was the daughter of the town's esteemed judge, known for her gentle demeanor and captivating smile. Thomas, on the other hand, was a charming young man who worked as a clerk in her father's courthouse.

Their paths crossed one fateful day when Emily's curiosity led her to wander into the courthouse, where Thomas was diligently organizing files. Their eyes met, and in that moment, something stirred within them – an unspoken connection that neither could deny.

As days passed, Emily found herself stealing glances at Thomas whenever she could, her heart fluttering like a trapped bird longing for freedom. And Thomas, though he tried to suppress his feelings, found himself drawn to Emily's grace and kindness.

Their secret glances soon turned into stolen conversations in the courthouse corridors, where they shared dreams and aspirations under the watchful gaze of Lady Justice, who seemed to smile upon their budding romance.

But their love was not without its challenges. Emily's father, Judge Anderson, held strict beliefs about social status and propriety, and the mere thought of his daughter falling for a humble clerk was enough to send shivers down his spine.

Despite the looming disapproval, Emily and Thomas continued to meet in secret, finding solace in each other's arms amidst the chaos of their forbidden love.

Then, one rainy afternoon, as they stood beneath the shelter of an old oak tree, Thomas gathered the courage to confess his love for Emily, his heart pounding with anticipation.

"I know we may never have the blessings of your father, but my love for you burns brighter than the sun," Thomas declared, his voice trembling with emotion.

Tears welled up in Emily's eyes as she reached out to caress his cheek, her love for him transcending the barriers of society. "And my heart belongs to you, Thomas, now and forever," she whispered, sealing their love with a tender kiss.

Their embrace was interrupted by the sound of footsteps approaching – Judge Anderson had discovered their secret rendezvous.

Faced with the disapproving gaze of her father, Emily stood tall, her love for Thomas unwavering. "Father, I know our love may seem unconventional, but it is real, and it is pure. Please, do not stand in the way of our happiness," she pleaded, her voice quivering with emotion.

For a moment, silence hung in the air like a heavy fog, until finally, Judge Anderson's stern expression softened, replaced by a glimmer of understanding.

In that moment, love triumphed over judgment, and as Emily and Thomas walked hand in hand into the sunset, they knew that their love was indeed a verdict worth fighting for.

# 36. Roxy's Rhapsody

In the vibrant streets of Chicago, where the rhythm of jazz filled the air like a sweet melody, lived two souls entwined in the world of music – Roxy and Joey.

Roxy was a talented singer, her voice like honey dripping from a golden comb, captivating all who heard her perform in the smoky jazz clubs of the city. Joey, a charismatic musician, was drawn to Roxy's enchanting voice like a sailor to the siren's song.

Their paths crossed one sultry summer night at a dimly lit jazz club, where Roxy's soulful rendition of "Summertime" cast a spell on Joey, leaving him spellbound and longing for more.

As they shared laughter and stories over glasses of bourbon, Joey found himself drawn to Roxy's warmth and passion, his heart skipping a beat whenever their eyes met across the crowded room.

But beneath the surface of their budding romance lurked the shadows of Joey's past – a past filled with broken promises and shattered dreams, a past he was desperate to leave behind.

As their love blossomed, Roxy found herself falling deeper and deeper for Joey, his charm and wit melting her heart like butter on a warm summer day. And Joey, unable to resist Roxy's allure, found himself torn between his desire for redemption and his fear of repeating past mistakes.

But fate had a way of testing their love, and soon, Joey's past came back to haunt him in the form of old debts and dangerous acquaintances, threatening to tear him away from Roxy's embrace.

Desperate to protect Roxy from the dangers of his world, Joey concocted a plan to leave Chicago and start anew, far away from the temptations that had led him astray.

But as he stood before Roxy, his heart heavy with guilt, he knew that he could not bear to leave her behind, his love for her burning brighter than any star in the night sky.

With tears streaming down his cheeks, Joey confessed his sins to Roxy, bracing himself for her inevitable rejection. But to his surprise, Roxy's reaction was not one of anger or disappointment, but of understanding and forgiveness.

"I may not be able to erase your past, Joey, but I believe in the power of redemption," Roxy whispered, her voice trembling with emotion. "And as long as we face the future together, I know we can overcome anything."

In that moment, Joey knew that he had found his salvation in Roxy's unwavering love, and as they embraced amidst the chaos of their lives, they vowed to build a future filled with music and laughter, leaving behind the shadows of Joey's past and embracing the promise of tomorrow.

## 37. Destiny's Stop

In the quiet town of Pleasantville, where the hum of everyday life echoed softly in the breeze, two souls found themselves intertwined in a journey of unexpected love – Glenda and John.

Glenda was a simple waitress at the local diner, her heart as warm as the coffee she served to weary travelers passing through town. John, a rugged cowboy with dreams as big as the endless sky, found himself stranded in Pleasantville when his bus broke down on its way to the next big rodeo.

Their paths crossed one rainy afternoon at the bus stop, where Glenda offered John a warm smile and a cup of hot coffee to chase away the chill of the storm. As they waited for the bus to be repaired, they shared stories and laughter, their connection growing stronger with each passing moment.

As the days turned into weeks, Glenda found herself drawn to John's rugged charm and unwavering determination, his presence bringing a spark of excitement to her otherwise ordinary life. And John, captivated by Glenda's kindness and sincerity, felt a longing in his heart he had never known before.

But their budding romance was not without its challenges. John's nomadic lifestyle clashed with

Glenda's desire for stability, and the looming reality of his departure weighed heavily on their hearts.

As they stood at the bus stop, their fingers intertwined like the intertwining branches of an old oak tree, John knew that he had to make a choice – to follow his dreams or to stay and build a future with Glenda by his side.

With a heavy heart, John boarded the bus bound for the next big rodeo, his mind filled with thoughts of Glenda and the love he left behind. And as the bus pulled away from the station, Glenda watched with tears in her eyes, her heart breaking with each passing mile.

But fate had other plans, and just when it seemed that their love was lost to the winds of time, John's bus broke down once again, this time just outside of Pleasantville.

With a sense of destiny guiding his steps, John returned to Glenda's side, his heart overflowing with love and determination. And as they stood together at the bus stop, their hands clasped tightly together, they knew that their love was worth waiting for, worth fighting for, no matter where the road may lead.

In the quiet town of Pleasantville, where the hum of everyday life echoed softly in the breeze, two souls found themselves intertwined in a journey of unexpected love – Glenda and John, bound together by the threads of fate and the promise of tomorrow.

## 38. Office Romance

In the bustling halls of the National Broadcasting Network, where the clatter of typewriters and the hum of telephones filled the air, two souls found themselves entangled in the whirlwind of office life – Betty and Tom.

Betty was the head of the reference department, known for her sharp wit and encyclopedic knowledge of facts and figures. Tom, a charming efficiency expert, was brought in to modernize the office and streamline its operations.

Their paths crossed one busy morning in the labyrinthine corridors of the office, where Betty's quick thinking and resourcefulness caught Tom's attention.

Intrigued by her intelligence and beauty, Tom found himself drawn to Betty like a moth to a flame.

As they worked together on various projects, Betty and Tom discovered a shared passion for problem-solving and a mutual respect for each other's abilities. Their professional relationship soon blossomed into friendship, and before long, they found themselves sharing lunches and laughter in the cozy confines of Betty's office.

But beneath the veneer of their professional rapport lurked the unspoken tension of burgeoning romance, a tension that neither Betty nor Tom could ignore.

As days turned into weeks and weeks turned into months, Betty and Tom found themselves dancing around the edges of something more, their hearts yearning to bridge the gap between friendship and love.

But the constraints of office politics and societal expectations threatened to keep them apart, casting a shadow over their budding romance.

Desperate to express his feelings, Tom devised a plan to woo Betty with grand gestures and romantic gestures, hoping to win her heart once and for all.

And so, on a crisp autumn evening, amidst the glow of candlelight and the soft strains of music, Tom confessed his love to Betty, his heart laid bare for her to see.

To his delight, Betty's response was not one of rejection or hesitation, but of joy and acceptance. "I've been waiting for you to say those words, Tom," she whispered, her eyes sparkling with emotion. "I love you too."

In that moment, surrounded by the warmth of their newfound love, Betty and Tom knew that their office romance was not just a fleeting infatuation, but a bond that would stand the test of time.

And as they embraced in the soft glow of the evening, they knew that their love story was just beginning, a tale of two hearts finding solace and companionship in the most unexpected of places – the bustling halls of the National Broadcasting Network.

# 39. Sweet Serenade

In the quaint neighborhood of Brookside, where the sound of laughter echoed through the streets like a symphony of joy, two hearts found solace and companionship in the melody of love – Sally and George.

Sally was the owner of the local music shop, her passion for melodies and harmonies evident in every note she played on her piano. George, a young musician with dreams of making it big in the jazz world, stumbled upon Sally's shop one sunny afternoon.

Their paths crossed amidst the rows of sheet music and gleaming instruments, where Sally's sweet smile and welcoming demeanor instantly captured George's heart. Entranced by her love for music and her gentle spirit, George found himself drawn to Sally like a moth to a flame.

As they spent time together, sharing stories and exchanging tunes, Sally and George discovered a shared passion for jazz and a deep connection that transcended words. Their love blossomed amidst the backdrop of music, each note serving as a testament to the beauty of their burgeoning romance.

But their happiness was not without its trials. George's pursuit of his dreams often took him away from Brookside, leaving Sally longing for his return and questioning the strength of their love.

Despite the distance, Sally remained steadfast in her belief in their love, her heart filled with hope and the promise of tomorrow.

And so, on a starlit evening beneath the swaying branches of an old oak tree, George serenaded Sally with a heartfelt melody, his love for her pouring forth in every chord and every note.

Touched by his sincerity and devotion, Sally knew that their love was as timeless as the songs they shared, a melody that would echo through the corridors of their hearts for eternity.

In that moment, surrounded by the soft glow of moonlight and the sweet strains of George's serenade,

Sally and George embraced, their love as pure and as beautiful as the music that brought them together.

And as they danced beneath the stars, lost in each other's arms, they knew that their love would endure, a sweet serenade that would never fade away.

## 40. Flames of Passion

In the lush jungles of Colombia, where the air was thick with the scent of tropical blooms and the sounds of exotic creatures, two hearts found themselves engulfed in the fiery embrace of passion – Elena and Diego.

Elena was a spirited botanist, her love for the vibrant flora of the jungle matched only by her fierce independence. Diego, a rugged adventurer with a penchant for danger, stumbled upon Elena's research camp one fateful day in search of emeralds rumored to lie hidden deep within the jungle.

Their paths crossed amidst the dense foliage and cascading waterfalls, where Elena's determination and beauty captivated Diego's heart like a moth to a flame.

Entranced by her fiery spirit and unwavering resolve, Diego found himself drawn to Elena in a way he had never experienced before.

As they ventured deeper into the heart of the jungle, Elena and Diego discovered a shared passion for adventure and a mutual respect for each other's abilities. Their days were filled with thrilling escapades and dangerous encounters, each moment bringing them closer together amidst the untamed beauty of the wilderness.

But their love was not without its challenges. The lure of emeralds and the dangers of the jungle threatened to tear them apart, casting a shadow over their budding romance.

Despite the obstacles they faced, Elena and Diego's love burned brighter than the green fire of the emeralds they sought, their hearts united in a bond as strong and enduring as the ancient trees that towered above them.

And so, amidst the flickering light of a campfire beneath the starlit sky, Diego declared his love for Elena, his words a testament to the depth of his passion and devotion.

Touched by his sincerity and unwavering love, Elena knew that their connection was as enduring as the green fire that glowed deep within the heart of the jungle, a flame that would never be extinguished.

In that moment, surrounded by the wild beauty of the Colombian wilderness, Elena and Diego embraced, their hearts aflame with the passion of a love that would withstand the test of time and the trials of the untamed jungle.

## 41. Harbor Serenade

In the picturesque coastal town of Harborview, where the salty sea air mingled with the sweet scent of blooming flowers, two hearts found themselves caught in the gentle ebb and flow of romance – Claire and Max.

Claire was a free-spirited artist, her paintings capturing the beauty of the seaside and the colors of the sunset.

Max, a handsome fisherman with a love for the ocean, stumbled upon Claire's art exhibition one sunny afternoon in the quaint town square.

Their paths crossed amidst the vibrant hues of Claire's paintings, where Max's admiration for her talent sparked a conversation that would change their lives forever.

"Your paintings are incredible," Max said, his eyes alight with genuine admiration as he examined Claire's artwork.

Blushing slightly, Claire smiled, her heart skipping a beat at the sight of Max's charming smile. "Thank you, Max. It means a lot coming from you."

Enchanted by her creativity and warmth, Max found himself drawn to Claire like a sailor to the call of the sea.

As they spent time together, exploring the hidden coves and sandy beaches of Harborview, Claire and Max discovered a shared love for the ocean and a mutual appreciation for the simple joys of life.

"Isn't the sunset breathtaking?" Claire exclaimed, her hand clasped in Max's as they watched the sun dip below the horizon, painting the sky in hues of pink and gold.

Max nodded, his gaze never leaving Claire's radiant smile. "It's even more beautiful with you by my side."

Their days were filled with laughter and adventure, each moment etched into their hearts like a seashell on the shore.

The whispers of gossip and the expectations of small-town life threatened to pull them apart, casting a shadow over their budding relationship.

Despite the obstacles they faced, Claire and Max's love for each other remained as steadfast as the tides, their hearts entwined in a bond as unbreakable as the waves crashing against the cliffs.

And so, on a balmy evening beneath the starlit sky, Max serenaded Claire with a heartfelt serenade, his guitar strumming softly as he poured out his feelings in song.

"Tears of joy filled Claire's eyes as she listened to Max's beautiful melody, her heart overflowing with love and gratitude.

"Touched by his sincerity and unwavering affection, Claire knew that their connection was as enduring as the ocean breeze that swept through their hair, a love that would weather any storm.

In that moment, surrounded by the beauty of nature and the sweet melody of Max's serenade, Claire and Max embraced, their hearts beating in rhythm with the pulse of the sea.

And as they walked hand in hand along the moonlit shore, they knew that their love was a treasure worth cherishing, a romance as timeless and beautiful as the coastal town of Harborview itself.

## 42. Starlight Serenade

In the dazzling world of Hollywood glamour, where the bright lights of fame shone like beacons in the night, two hearts found themselves swept away by the magic of stardom and romance – Ava and James.

Ava was a talented aspiring actress, her beauty and grace capturing the attention of casting directors and producers alike. James, a charming photographer with a passion for capturing the essence of beauty, stumbled upon Ava's audition one fateful day in the bustling streets of Hollywood.

Their paths crossed amidst the glitz and glamour of the studio lot, where Ava's captivating audition caught James' eye like a shooting star in the night sky. Enchanted by her talent and presence, James found himself drawn to Ava like a moth to a flame.

As they spent time together on set, capturing Ava's beauty through his lens, Ava and James discovered a shared passion for the art of filmmaking and a mutual admiration for each other's talents. Their days were filled with laughter and excitement, each moment tinged with the promise of stardom and success.

Amidst the allure of Hollywood's glittering facade, Ava and James faced their share of hurdles. The pressures of

Hollywood and the allure of fame threatened to pull them apart, casting a shadow over their budding relationship.

Despite the obstacles they faced, Ava and James' love for each other remained as bright as the stars that adorned the Hollywood sky, their hearts entwined in a bond as unbreakable as the silver screen.

And so, on a starry night beneath the glimmering lights of the studio lot, James serenaded Ava with a heartfelt serenade, his camera capturing the magic of their love in every frame.

"Touched by his sincerity and unwavering affection, Ava knew that their connection was as enduring as the Hollywood stars that watched over them, a love that would withstand the test of time.

In that moment, surrounded by the beauty of the silver screen and the sweet melody of James' serenade, Ava and James embraced, their hearts beating in rhythm with the pulse of the city.

And as they walked hand in hand along the starlit boulevard, they knew that their love was a story worth telling, a romance as timeless and beautiful as the movies themselves.

## 43. A Serendipitous Affair

In the vibrant streets of San Francisco, where the city's heartbeat echoed through the bustling crowds, two souls found themselves drawn together in the delight of each other's presence – Emily and Daniel.

Emily was a lively socialite, her laughter like music in the air as she charmed her way through elegant soirées and glamorous gatherings. Daniel, a worldly gentleman with a penchant for adventure, crossed paths with Emily at a charity event one enchanting evening.

Their meeting sparked an instant connection, as Emily's vivacious spirit captivated Daniel, drawing him into her world with effortless grace and charm.

As they spent time together, exploring the city's hidden gems and indulging in lively conversation, Emily and

Daniel discovered a shared appreciation for life's pleasures and a mutual admiration for each other's company.

"I must say, Emily, your knowledge of the city's history is quite impressive," Daniel remarked, his eyes twinkling with admiration as they strolled along the waterfront.

"Oh, Daniel, you flatter me," Emily replied with a playful smile. "But I must admit, it's easy to be enthusiastic about San Francisco when I'm in such delightful company."

Their days were filled with laughter and excitement, each moment an affirmation of the joy they found in each other's presence.

Despite the challenges they faced, Emily and Daniel's bond continued to deepen, their connection growing stronger with each passing day.

And so, amidst the vibrant energy of the city, Daniel serenaded Emily with tales of his adventures and dreams, his words a testament to the depth of his affection.

"Touched by his sincerity and the pleasure of his company, Emily knew that their connection was something truly special, a bond that transcended time and distance."

In that moment, surrounded by the beauty of San Francisco's skyline and the warmth of Daniel's embrace, Emily and Daniel embraced, their hearts united in a shared journey of love and discovery.

And as they walked hand in hand through the city streets, they knew that their love was a treasure worth cherishing, a serendipitous affair that would light their way through life's adventures.

## 44. A Little Bit of Love

In the heart of a bustling city lived a young woman named Judith. She worked in a quaint bookstore nestled between towering buildings. Her days were filled with the smell of old books and the sound of pages turning. But beneath her quiet exterior, she harbored dreams of adventure and romance.

One day, while organizing the shelves, Judith stumbled upon a peculiar book. Its cover was worn, and its pages seemed to whisper secrets of love. Curiosity piqued, she opened it to find a note tucked inside. It read, "Find love where you least expect it."

Determined to uncover the mystery behind the note, Judith embarked on a journey to explore the city. Along the way, she encountered a charming young man named Alex, who worked as a photographer for a local magazine. His easy smile and adventurous spirit captured Judith's heart.

As they spent more time together, Judith and Alex discovered shared interests and dreams. They laughed under the city lights, danced in the rain, and shared whispered secrets beneath the stars. With each passing day, their bond grew stronger, and love blossomed between them.

But amidst their newfound happiness, challenges arose. Alex's demanding job often kept him away for days at a time, leaving Judith longing for his presence. And as they navigated the complexities of their relationship, doubts and insecurities crept in.

Yet, through it all, Judith and Alex remained steadfast in their love for each other. They learned to cherish every moment they shared, knowing that love was worth fighting for. And as they embraced the unpredictability of life, they realized that sometimes, the greatest adventures are found in the arms of the ones we love.

In the end, Judith and Alex's love story was not without its twists and turns. But through laughter and tears, they discovered that true love knows no bounds. And as they walked hand in hand through the city streets, they knew that their journey was only just beginning.

For Judith and Alex, the pages of their love story were filled with endless possibilities. And as they faced each new chapter together, they knew that as long as they had each other, they could live a little and love a little more.

# 45. A Swing of Love

In a small town nestled amidst rolling hills lived a young woman named Betty. She was known for her prowess on the tennis court, where her powerful strokes and graceful movements mesmerized spectators. But beneath her athletic exterior, Betty harbored a secret longing for something more.

One sunny afternoon, as Betty practiced her serves at the local tennis club, she caught the eye of a charming young man named Bobby. He was a coach from the nearby city, drawn to Betty's natural talent and undeniable charm. Their eyes met across the court, and in that moment, a spark ignited between them.

"Nice swing, Betty," Bobby said, flashing her a grin as she hit a perfect forehand.

"Thanks, Bobby," Betty replied, feeling her cheeks flush with warmth. "You're not too bad yourself."

As Betty and Bobby spent more time together, their connection deepened. They shared laughter and stories, dreams and aspirations. Bobby admired Betty's determination and drive, while Betty found solace in Bobby's unwavering support and encouragement.

But their budding romance was not without its obstacles. Betty's strict coach, Mr. Thompson, disapproved of her relationship with Bobby, fearing it would distract her from her training. And as Betty struggled to balance her passion for tennis with her newfound love, doubts and insecurities crept in.

"I don't know if I can do this, Bobby," Betty confessed one evening, her voice tinged with uncertainty.

Bobby took her hand in his, his gaze unwavering. "You can do anything you set your mind to, Betty. I believe in you."

Yet, despite the challenges they faced, Betty and Bobby remained steadfast in their love for each other. They found strength in each other's arms, and courage in each other's words. And as they navigated the highs and lows of their relationship, they discovered that love was worth fighting for.

In the end, Betty's determination paid off, as she triumphed on the tennis court and in matters of the heart. With Bobby by her side, she soared to new heights, both in her sport and in her personal life. And as they celebrated their victories together, they knew that their love was a match made in heaven.

For Betty and Bobby, their romance was like a perfect serve, precise and powerful, with just the right amount of spin. And as they looked towards the future, hand in hand, they knew that together, they could conquer anything that came their way.

In the quaint town where they first met, Betty and Bobby's love story became the talk of the town. And as they exchanged vows under the clear blue sky, surrounded by family and friends, they knew that their love was destined to last a lifetime.

For Betty and Bobby, love was not just a game—it was a swing of destiny. And as they embarked on this new chapter of their lives together, they knew that their love would only continue to grow stronger with each passing day.

# 46. The Society Scandal

In the affluent suburbs of Philadelphia, amidst the grandeur of sprawling estates and lavish parties, lived a young socialite named Katherine. She was the epitome of grace and elegance, admired by all who knew her. But beneath her polished exterior, Katherine harbored a secret longing for freedom and independence.

One evening, as Katherine prepared for yet another extravagant soiree, she received an unexpected visit from her ex-husband, Charles. He was a charming and witty man, with a knack for stirring up trouble wherever he went. Their past was filled with tumultuous ups and downs, yet there remained an undeniable spark between them.

"Katherine, my dear, you look as radiant as ever," Charles remarked, his smile as disarming as ever.

Katherine arched an eyebrow, her demeanor cool and collected. "What brings you here, Charles? Surely you haven't come to crash another one of my parties."

As they exchanged barbs and banter, Katherine and Charles found themselves drawn back into the familiar dance of their past. Despite their differences, there was an undeniable chemistry between them—a connection that refused to be ignored.

Their reunion was not so easy. Katherine was set to marry her fiancé, George, a respectable and dependable man who offered her security and stability. And as she grappled with her feelings for Charles, Katherine found herself torn between the expectations of society and the desires of her heart.

"I never thought I'd see you again, Katherine," Charles admitted one evening, his voice tinged with vulnerability.

Katherine sighed, her gaze lingering on the man she once loved. "Nor did I, Charles. But some things are simply meant to be."

As Katherine navigated the intricacies of her complicated love life, she found herself questioning the choices she had made. Was she willing to sacrifice her own happiness for the sake of societal approval? Or would she have the courage to follow her heart, no matter the consequences?

In the end, Katherine's journey led her to a revelation—a realization that true love could not be confined by the constraints of social status or expectation. With Charles by her side, she embraced the freedom to be herself, unapologetically and unabashedly.

In the elite circles of Philadelphia society, Katherine and Charles's romance became the talk of the town—a scandalous affair that defied all expectations. And as they faced the judgmental glances and disapproving whispers, they stood tall, secure in the knowledge that their love was stronger than any societal convention.

For Katherine and Charles, The Society Scandal was not just a chapter in their lives—it was a love story for the ages, destined to be remembered long after the last champagne glass had been emptied and the final guest had bid farewell.

# 47. G.I. Love on Leave

In the bustling streets of West Germany, amidst the vibrant energy of post-war reconstruction, lived a young soldier named Johnny. He was a G.I. stationed at a nearby military base, his days filled with drills and duties. But beneath his uniform, Johnny harbored dreams of music and romance.

One evening, as Johnny and his fellow soldiers enjoyed a night out on the town, they stumbled upon a lively nightclub where the sound of jazz filled the air. It was there that Johnny first laid eyes on a captivating young woman named Lisa. She was a singer with a voice like velvet, her presence commanding the attention of everyone in the room.

"Hey there, soldier boy," Lisa greeted Johnny with a playful smile as he approached the stage.

Johnny grinned, his heart racing with excitement. "Evening, miss. Mind if I join you for a dance?"

As they swayed to the rhythm of the music, Johnny and Lisa discovered a shared love for song and dance. They laughed and talked late into the night, their connection growing stronger with each passing moment. Despite the uncertainty of their futures, they found solace in each other's company, cherishing the fleeting moments they shared.

Johnny's impending deployment loomed large, casting a shadow over their newfound love. And as they grappled with the reality of their situation, doubts and insecurities threatened to tear them apart.

"I don't know how we'll make it work, Johnny," Lisa confessed one evening, her voice tinged with sadness.

Johnny pulled her close, his embrace offering comfort and reassurance. "We'll find a way, Lisa. I promise."

Together, Johnny and Lisa navigated the challenges of a long-distance romance, their love sustaining them through the trials of separation. They wrote letters and exchanged tokens of affection, counting down the days until they could be reunited once more.

In the end, Johnny's tour of duty came to an end, and he returned to West Germany with a newfound appreciation for the things that truly mattered. With Lisa by his side, he embarked on a new chapter of his life, filled with hope and possibility.

For Johnny and Lisa, Love on Leave was not just a fleeting romance—it was a bond forged in the fires of adversity, a love that endured despite the odds. And as they looked towards the future, hand in hand, they knew that their love would only continue to grow stronger with each passing day.

## 48. The Unwavering Molly Jones

In the bustling city of Denver, amidst the rugged beauty of the Rocky Mountains, lived a spirited young woman named Molly. She was a force to be reckoned with—a trailblazer and a pioneer in her own right. But beneath her fiery exterior, Molly harbored dreams of a life filled with adventure and excitement.

One fateful day, as Molly boarded a steamboat bound for the bustling port city of St. Louis, she found herself swept up in a whirlwind romance with a charming young man named Charlie. He was a dashing prospector with dreams of striking it rich in the gold mines of the West. Their paths crossed unexpectedly, setting the stage for an unforgettable journey.

"Mind if I join you, miss?" Charlie asked with a twinkle in his eye as Molly settled into her seat on the deck of the steamboat.

Molly flashed him a grin, her spirit as indomitable as ever. "Not at all, stranger. But fair warning—I'm not one for idle chatter."

As they sailed down the mighty Mississippi River, Molly and Charlie discovered a shared love for adventure and a thirst for the unknown. They laughed and danced beneath the stars, their hearts beating in time with the rhythm of the river. Despite the challenges that lay ahead, they found solace in each other's company, united by a sense of purpose and determination.

Their journey was to have some surprises. Along the way, they faced treacherous rapids, fierce storms, and the ever-present threat of danger lurking around every bend in the river. Yet, through it all, Molly and Charlie remained undeterred, their love for each other guiding them through even the darkest of times.

"I never expected to find love on the river," Molly confessed one evening, her voice soft against the backdrop of the setting sun.

Charlie reached out to take her hand, his touch warm and reassuring. "Nor did I, Molly. But sometimes, the best things in life come when you least expect them."

Together, Molly and Charlie braved the challenges of the river, their love growing stronger with each passing day. And as they reached the bustling port city of St. Louis, they knew that their journey was far from over. With hearts full of hope and a sense of adventure burning bright, they set out to conquer the world together, one daring escapade at a time.

For Molly and Charlie, The Unwavering Molly Jones was not just a tale of love—it was about the power of resilience and determination in the face of adversity. And as they charted their course through life's uncertain waters, they did so with unwavering faith in each other and the unshakeable belief that together, they could overcome any obstacle that came their way.

## 49. Royal Serenade of Love

In the opulent halls of a European palace, amidst the grandeur of ballrooms and sweeping gardens, lived a young princess named Anna. She was the epitome of grace and beauty, admired by all who knew her. But beneath her regal exterior, Anna longed for a love that transcended the confines of duty and tradition.

One fateful day, as Anna attended a royal gala, she caught the eye of a dashing young prince named Edward. He was a nobleman from a neighboring kingdom, his charm and wit captivating all who crossed his path. Their meeting sparked a whirlwind romance that would forever change the course of their lives.

"May I have this dance, Your Highness?" Edward asked, extending his hand to Anna with a smile.

Anna's heart skipped a beat as she placed her hand in his, her cheeks flushed with excitement. "I would be honored, Your Grace."

As they danced beneath the shimmering chandeliers, Anna and Edward discovered a connection that went beyond the boundaries of their royal status. They laughed and talked late into the night, their souls entwined in a serenade of love that echoed through the halls of the palace.

But there was trouble looming. Anna's parents, the king and queen, had already arranged a political marriage for her—a union that would secure an alliance between their kingdoms. And as Anna and Edward navigated the treacherous waters of court intrigue and familial duty, they found themselves torn between their love for each other and their obligations to their respective kingdoms.

"I cannot bear the thought of living without you, Anna," Edward confessed one evening, his voice filled with anguish.

Anna reached out to take his hand, her eyes brimming with tears. "Nor can I, Edward. But we cannot defy our families and the traditions that bind us."

Together, Anna and Edward faced the challenges that threatened to tear them apart, their love for each other shining bright even in the darkest of times. And as they stood on the precipice of a future filled with uncertainty, they knew that their love was worth fighting for, no matter the cost.

In the end, Anna and Edward's love prevailed against all odds. With courage in their hearts and determination in their souls, they forged a path forward together, united in their commitment to each other and the promise of a future filled with hope and happiness.

For Anna and Edward, Serenade of Love was not just a fleeting romance—it was a testament to the power of love to conquer all obstacles and defy the expectations of society. And as they walked hand in hand into the sunset, their hearts full of joy and their spirits soaring high, they knew that their love would endure for all eternity.

# 50. Wings of Destiny

In the rugged landscape of a South American port town, where the skies were as unpredictable as the hearts of its inhabitants, lived a group of daring aviators known as the Flying Braves. They were a band of fearless pilots, risking their lives day in and day out to navigate the treacherous skies and deliver cargo to remote locations. But beneath their bravado and swagger, each pilot carried the weight of their own past and the scars of their own experiences.

One stormy evening, as the pilots gathered at their favorite watering hole, they encountered a mysterious woman named Nora. She was a stranger to the town, her presence as enigmatic as the storm clouds gathering overhead. And as Nora shared her own tales of adventure and hardship, she found herself drawn to the camaraderie and courage of the Flying Braves.

"Quite a storm we've got brewing," one of the pilots remarked, his voice tinged with anticipation.

Nora nodded, her eyes gleaming with excitement. "I've always been drawn to the thrill of the unknown."

As the storm raged on outside, the pilots and Nora forged a bond that transcended the boundaries of friendship and adventure. They laughed and joked, sharing stories of their daring exploits and narrow escapes. And as the night wore on, they found themselves drawn closer together, united by a shared sense of purpose and a longing for something more.

But their newfound camaraderie was put to the test when tragedy struck, and one of their own fell victim to the unforgiving skies. As the pilots grappled with their grief and guilt, Nora stood by their side, offering comfort and support in their darkest hour.

"I never expected to find a family among a group of daredevils," Nora confessed one evening, her voice soft against the backdrop of the howling wind.

One of the pilots reached out to take her hand, his touch gentle and reassuring. "Nor did we, Nora. But sometimes, the bonds we form in the face of danger are the strongest of all."

Together, the Flying Braves and Nora faced the challenges of their precarious existence, their bond growing stronger with each passing day. And as they soared through the skies, navigating the storms of life with courage and determination, they knew that their destiny was written in the stars.

## 51. Lessons in Love

In the bustling halls of a prestigious university, amidst the eager minds and scholarly pursuits, lived a passionate young journalist named Laura. She was a woman ahead of her time, determined to make her mark in a world dominated by men. But beneath her fierce exterior, Laura harbored doubts about her own abilities and a longing for acceptance and recognition.

One day, as Laura attended a lecture on journalism, she found herself drawn to the charismatic professor, Michael. He was a seasoned journalist with a wealth of experience and wisdom, his passion for the craft evident in every word he spoke. Their meeting sparked a connection that transcended the boundaries of academia, setting the stage for an unexpected romance.

"Your insights on investigative reporting are truly inspiring, Professor," Laura remarked, her voice filled with admiration.

Michael smiled, his eyes twinkling with amusement. "Why, thank you, Miss Laura. I must say, I'm equally impressed by your enthusiasm for the subject."

As they delved deeper into the world of journalism together, Laura and Michael discovered a shared passion for truth and integrity. They debated ethics and debated ethics, challenged each other's perspectives, and found solace in the company of someone who shared their values and aspirations.

However, Laura struggled to balance her newfound feelings for Michael with her desire to prove herself in a male-dominated field. And Michael, haunted by the ghosts of his past, grappled with his own insecurities and fears of commitment.

"I never expected to fall for my professor," Laura confessed one evening, her voice tinged with vulnerability.

Michael reached out to take her hand, his touch gentle and reassuring. "Nor did I, Laura. But sometimes, love finds us in the most unexpected of places."

Together, Laura and Michael navigated the complexities of their relationship, confronting their fears and insecurities head-on. And as they embarked on a journey of self-discovery and growth, they discovered that true love was not about perfection, but about acceptance and understanding.

In the end, Laura and Michael's love prevailed against all odds. With courage in their hearts and a shared commitment to honesty and integrity, they forged a path forward together, leaving behind the doubts and insecurities that had held them back.

For Laura and Michael, Lessons in Love was not just a romance—it was a journey of self-discovery and growth, a testament to the transformative power of love to heal old wounds and illuminate the path to a brighter future. And as they walked hand in hand into the unknown, their hearts full of hope and their spirits soaring high, they knew that their love would endure, a beacon of hope in a world filled with uncertainty.

## 52. The Royal Encounter

In the grandeur of 1950s London, amidst the glitz and glamour of the theater world, lived a young actress named Alice. She was a rising star, her talent captivating audiences and drawing the attention of critics and admirers alike. But beneath her poised exterior, Alice yearned for a love that transcended the superficiality of fame and fortune.

One fateful day, as Alice prepared for her latest performance, she caught the eye of a charming young prince named Edward. He was a member of European royalty, his presence commanding attention wherever he went. Their meeting sparked a whirlwind romance that would forever change the course of their lives.

"Your performance was simply captivating, Miss Alice," Edward remarked, his voice filled with admiration.

Alice blushed, her heart fluttering at the prince's praise. "Thank you, Your Highness. It's an honor to have you in the audience."

As they spent more time together, Alice and Edward discovered a shared love for the arts and a longing for a connection that went beyond the constraints of their respective worlds. They laughed and talked late into the night, their hearts entwined in a dance of passion and desire.

As time passed, Alice struggled to reconcile her newfound feelings for Edward with the pressures of her career and the expectations placed upon her by society. And Edward, torn between duty and desire, grappled with the weight of his royal responsibilities and the dictates of his heart.

"I never expected to find love in the arms of an actress," Edward confessed one evening, his voice tinged with uncertainty.

Alice reached out to take his hand, her touch gentle and reassuring. "Nor did I, Edward. But sometimes, love knows no bounds."

Together, Alice and Edward navigated the complexities of their relationship, facing obstacles and opposition from those who sought to keep them apart. But with each challenge they encountered, their love only grew stronger, fueled by the depth of their connection and the intensity of their emotions.

In the end, Alice and Edward's love prevailed against all odds. With courage in their hearts and a shared commitment to each other, they forged a path forward together, leaving behind the constraints of their pasts and embracing a future filled with hope and possibility.

## 53. Love in Disguise

In the bustling streets of 1960s New York City, amidst the hustle and bustle of daily life, lived a young woman named Emily. She was a dedicated nurse, her days spent caring for those in need with unwavering compassion and dedication. But beneath her professional demeanor, Emily harbored a secret longing for a life filled with adventure and romance.

One fateful day, as Emily tended to her patients at the local hospital, she crossed paths with a charming young doctor named Matthew. He was a newcomer to the city, his presence bringing a breath of fresh air to the hospital wards. Their meeting sparked a connection that transcended the confines of their professional roles, setting the stage for an unexpected romance.

"Your dedication to your patients is truly inspiring, Miss Emily," Matthew remarked, his eyes filled with admiration.

Emily blushed, her heart fluttering at the doctor's praise. "Thank you, Doctor Matthew. It's all in a day's work."

As they worked side by side, Emily and Matthew discovered a shared passion for healing and a desire to make a difference in the world. They laughed and talked late into the night, their bond growing stronger with each passing day. But their budding romance was not without its challenges.

Emily struggled to balance her responsibilities as a nurse with her growing feelings for Matthew, while Matthew grappled with the demands of his career and the expectations placed upon him by his colleagues. And as they navigated the complexities of their relationship, they found themselves drawn deeper into a web of secrecy and deception.

"I never expected to find love in the halls of a hospital," Matthew confessed one evening, his voice filled with uncertainty.

Emily reached out to take his hand, her touch gentle and reassuring. "Nor did I, Matthew. But sometimes, love comes when we least expect it, in the most unlikely of places."

Together, Emily and Matthew faced the challenges of their relationship head-on, confronting their fears and insecurities with honesty and courage. And as they embarked on a journey of self-discovery and growth, they discovered that true love was worth any sacrifice.

In the end, Emily and Matthew's love prevailed against all odds. With courage in their hearts and a shared commitment to each other, they forged a path forward together, leaving behind the shadows of their pasts and embracing a future filled with hope and possibility.

## 54. Heartstrings Melody

In the tranquil countryside of 1950s Tennessee, where the air was filled with the sweet scent of magnolias and the sound of gentle breezes rustling through the trees, lived a young woman named Mary. She was a vision of innocence and grace, her heart as pure as the dew-kissed petals of a rose. But beneath her demure exterior, Mary harbored dreams of a love that would sweep her off her feet and carry her to new heights of happiness.

One fateful day, as Mary tended to her family's farm, she crossed paths with a rugged young soldier named James. He was a recent returnee from the Civil War, his eyes haunted by the memories of battle and loss. Their meeting sparked a connection that would forever change the course of their lives.

"Your kindness is like a ray of sunshine on a cloudy day, Miss Mary," James remarked, his voice tinged with gratitude.

Mary smiled, her heart fluttering at the soldier's words. "It's the least I can do to thank you for your service, Mr. James. You've sacrificed so much for our country."

As they worked side by side on the farm, Mary and James discovered a shared love for the land and a longing for a future filled with peace and prosperity. They laughed and talked late into the night, their bond growing stronger with each passing day. But their budding romance was not without its challenges.

James struggled to come to terms with the horrors of war and the scars it had left on his soul, while Mary grappled with the expectations of her family and the constraints of her rural upbringing. And as they navigated the complexities of their relationship, they found themselves drawn deeper into a web of love and longing.

"I never expected to find love in the aftermath of war," James confessed one evening, his voice filled with wonder.

"Nor did I, James. But sometimes, love blooms in the most unexpected of places, like a wildflower in a field of green," she tenderly replied.

Together, Mary and James faced the challenges of their relationship with courage and determination, their love shining bright even in the darkest of times. And as they embraced the promise of a future filled with hope and possibility, they knew that their love was worth any sacrifice.

In the end, Mary and James's love prevailed against all odds. With hearts full of joy and a steadfast commitment to each other, they forged a path forward together, leaving behind the shadows of their pasts and embracing a future filled with love and laughter.

# 55. Harbor of Hearts

In the quaint fishing village of Marseille, nestled along the sun-kissed shores of the French Riviera, lived a spirited young woman named Isabelle, affectionately known as Fanny. She was the heart and soul of the seaside community, her laughter echoing through the cobbled streets and her kindness touching the lives of all who knew her. But beneath her carefree exterior, Fanny harbored a secret longing for a love that would sweep her off her feet and carry her away to distant shores.

One fateful day, as Fanny tended to her family's bustling seafood restaurant, she crossed paths with a charming sailor named André. He was a rugged and enigmatic figure, his eyes sparkling with a sense of adventure and mystery. Their meeting sparked a connection that would forever change the course of their lives.

"Your smile is like a ray of sunshine on a cloudy day, Mademoiselle Fanny," André remarked, his voice tinged with admiration.

Fanny blushed, her heart fluttering at the sailor's compliment. "Merci, Monsieur André. You have a way with words."

As they spent more time together, Fanny and André discovered a shared love for the sea and a longing for a life filled with romance and adventure. They laughed and talked late into the night, their bond growing stronger with each passing day. But their budding romance was not without its challenges.

Fanny struggled to reconcile her feelings for André with the expectations of her family and the responsibilities of her upbringing. And André, haunted by the memories of his past and the fear of commitment, grappled with his own doubts and insecurities. Yet, despite the obstacles that stood in their way, Fanny and André found themselves drawn deeper into a whirlwind of passion and desire.

"I never expected to find love in a small fishing village," André confessed one evening, his voice filled with wonder.

Fanny reached out to take his hand, her touch gentle and reassuring. "Nor did I, André. But sometimes, love washes ashore when we least expect it, like a treasure hidden beneath the waves."

Together, Fanny and André embarked on a journey of self-discovery and growth, their love shining bright even in the darkest of times. And as they embraced the promise of a future filled with hope and possibility, they knew that their love was worth any sacrifice.

In the end, Fanny and André's love prevailed against all odds. With hearts full of joy and a steadfast commitment to each other, they forged a path forward together, leaving behind the doubts and insecurities that had held them back.

## 56. Summer Serenade

In the quaint town of Seabreeze, where the sun danced on the waves and laughter filled the air, lived two souls destined to collide: Molly and Jack.

Molly, with her fiery spirit and heart as vast as the ocean, worked at the local diner, serving up smiles along with milkshakes. Jack, a charming musician with a guitar for a heart, strummed melodies that echoed through the streets.

Their paths crossed one balmy summer evening at the town's annual beach bonfire. Underneath the star-studded sky, Jack's fingers danced on the strings, serenading the crowd with sweet tunes. Molly, captivated by his music, found herself drawn to him like a moth to a flame.

As the night wore on, they found themselves lost in conversation, sharing dreams and aspirations under the moon's gentle glow. With each word exchanged, an invisible thread wove itself between their hearts, binding them in an unspoken promise of something more.

Days turned into nights, and nights turned into stolen moments shared on sandy shores and hidden coves. With each passing sunrise, their bond deepened, blossoming like the wildflowers that adorned the cliffs overlooking the sea.

But as summer waned and the days grew shorter, a shadow loomed on the horizon. Jack's impending departure weighed heavy on their hearts, casting a bittersweet hue over their stolen moments of bliss.

In a desperate attempt to hold onto the fleeting magic of their summer romance, Molly and Jack embarked on a whirlwind adventure, exploring every corner of their seaside haven and savoring each precious moment together.

As the final days of summer slipped through their fingers like grains of sand, Molly and Jack found themselves standing at the edge of the ocean, the waves whispering secrets of love lost and dreams deferred.

With tears in her eyes and a tremble in her voice, Molly whispered a promise into the salty breeze, vowing to carry their love with her wherever she roamed. And as Jack boarded the train bound for distant shores, he turned to her with a smile that spoke volumes, knowing that their love would endure, no matter the distance between them.

And so, as the sun set on their summer romance, Molly and Jack parted ways, their hearts forever intertwined, their souls bound by the timeless melody of love. For in the end, they knew that true love knows no bounds, and that no distance could ever dim the flame that burned between them.

## 57. A Flight of Hearts

In the bustling halls of London's Heathrow Airport, where dreams took flight and hearts soared, fate weaved its intricate web, entangling the lives of two strangers: Emily and David.

Emily, a radiant beauty with a heart as vast as the sky, stood amidst the hustle and bustle, her eyes shimmering with anticipation as she awaited her departure to distant lands. David, a suave businessman with a magnetic charm, found himself stranded in the airport lounge, his plans derailed by unforeseen circumstances.

As fate would have it, their paths crossed in the most unexpected of ways. Drawn together by a chance encounter, Emily and David found themselves embarking on a journey that would forever alter the course of their lives.

Amidst the chaos of delayed flights and missed connections, a bond began to form between them, forged in the crucible of shared laughter and stolen glances. With each passing moment, they found solace in each other's company, finding refuge from the storm raging outside within the sanctuary of their shared connection.

As the hours stretched into eternity, Emily and David found themselves ensnared in a whirlwind of emotions, their hearts laid bare amidst the sterile confines of the airport lounge. In each other's arms, they discovered a kindred spirit, a soulmate whose presence filled the void in their hearts with a warmth that defied explanation.

As the clock ticked relentlessly towards their inevitable parting, reality came crashing down around them, threatening to shatter the fragile bubble of their newfound love. With Emily's departure imminent, David found himself torn between duty and desire, his heart torn asunder by the prospect of losing her forever.

In a desperate bid to seize the moment, David threw caution to the wind, declaring his love for Emily in a passionate outpouring of emotion that echoed through the empty corridors of the airport. And as Emily gazed into his eyes, she knew in that moment that she had found her true North, her guiding light amidst the darkness of uncertainty.

With their hearts entwined in a love that transcended time and space, Emily and David embraced beneath the flickering lights of the departure lounge, vowing to defy the odds and overcome whatever obstacles stood in their way. For in each other's arms, they had found a refuge from the storms of life, a sanctuary where their love could take flight and soar to new heights.

## 58. A Physician's Predicament

In the hallowed halls of a prestigious London hospital, where lives hung in the balance and the weight of responsibility bore down on weary shoulders, one doctor found himself torn between duty and desire: Dr. Robert and Dr. Elizabeth.

Dr. Robert, a brilliant physician with a heart as compassionate as it was conflicted, dedicated his life to the service of others, tirelessly striving to heal the sick and mend broken bodies. Dr. Elizabeth, a talented surgeon with a sharp mind and a gentle touch, shared his passion for medicine and his unwavering commitment to his patients.

Their paths crossed one fateful day in the operating room, where they worked side by side, their hands steady and their minds sharp as they fought to save the lives entrusted to their care. In each other's presence, they found a kindred spirit, a soulmate whose passion for healing mirrored their own.

As they navigated the complexities of their profession, Dr. Robert and Dr. Elizabeth found themselves drawn together by an undeniable attraction that transcended the boundaries of professionalism. With each passing day, their bond deepened, until they found themselves teetering on the brink of something more than just friendship.

As the demands of their profession threatened to consume them, Dr. Robert and Dr. Elizabeth found themselves faced with an impossible choice: to follow the dictates of their hearts and risk their careers, or to suppress their feelings and maintain the facade of professionalism.

In the end, it was love that triumphed over duty, a love as pure and true as the Hippocratic oath itself. With courage in their hearts and determination in their souls, Dr. Robert and Dr. Elizabeth cast aside the shackles of propriety and embraced their destiny, their love a testament to the healing power of the human heart.

# 59. Echoes in Africa

In the vast expanse of the African wilderness, where the snow-capped peaks of Kilimanjaro loomed like silent sentinels over the savannah below, two souls found themselves confronting the ghosts of their past and the fleeting beauty of the present: Helen and David.

"Helen, look at that," David said, his voice hushed with awe as he pointed towards the majestic mountain rising into the night sky.

Helen's eyes widened in wonder as she followed his gaze. "It's breathtaking, David," she whispered, her voice filled with reverence. "I've never seen anything like it."

Bound together by a shared sense of wanderlust and a longing for redemption, they embarked on a journey of self-discovery and reflection, their hearts intertwined like the roots of the ancient baobab trees that dotted the landscape.

As they traversed the rugged terrain of the African wilderness, Helen and David confronted the demons of their pasts and the regrets that threatened to consume them whole. With each step forward, they found solace in the beauty of the natural world around them, their bond deepening with every shared moment of awe and wonder.

"In all my years of travel, I've never felt as alive as I do right now," Helen said, her voice tinged with emotion as she looked into David's eyes.

David nodded, his own eyes reflecting the fire burning within his soul. "Neither have I, Helen. It's like every step we take brings us closer to something greater than ourselves."

In a moment of raw honesty and vulnerability, Helen and David laid bare their souls to each other, their hearts laid bare beneath the endless expanse of the African sky. With the snows of Kilimanjaro as their witness and the whispers of the wind as their guide, they embraced the beauty of the present and the promise of a future filled with endless possibility.

## 60. The Reporter's Rendezvous

In the bustling newsroom of the Morning Herald, where the clatter of typewriters and the hum of telephone lines filled the air with a symphony of chaos, two relentless journalists found themselves caught in the whirlwind of breaking news and rekindled romance: Rosie and Jack.

Rosie, a tenacious reporter with a quick wit and a knack for getting to the heart of the story, had left the fast-paced world of journalism behind to pursue a quieter life. Jack, her former editor and ex-husband, was a seasoned newsman with a nose for a scoop and a reputation for stirring up trouble wherever he went.

Their paths collided one fateful day when Jack walked back into the newsroom, his presence sending shockwaves through the staff and setting the stage for a reunion neither of them expected. Drawn together by the irresistible pull of their shared past and the thrill of the chase, they found themselves embroiled in a high-stakes game of journalistic intrigue and romantic tension.

As they raced against the clock to break the story of a lifetime, Rosie and Jack found themselves grappling with the ghosts of their failed marriage and the unresolved feelings that still lingered between them. With each heated exchange and stolen moment of intimacy, they were forced to confront the truth of their own hearts and the undeniable chemistry that still simmered beneath the surface.

But as the deadline loomed and the pressure mounted, Rosie and Jack found themselves faced with an impossible choice: to follow their heads and pursue the story, or to listen to their hearts and give love a second chance. With the fate of their careers and their hearts hanging in the balance, they embarked on a whirlwind adventure that would test the limits of their resolve and redefine the meaning of true love.

In a moment of reckless abandon, Rosie and Jack threw caution to the wind and surrendered to the undeniable pull of their passion, their hearts soaring as they embraced the thrill of the chase and the promise of a future together. With the newsroom buzzing with excitement and the city streets alive with the rhythm of their love, they knew that they had finally found their happy ending in each other's arms.

And as they walked hand in hand into the sunset, their laughter ringing out like a clarion call to all who dared to dream, Rosie and Jack knew that their love was a story for the ages, a testament to the enduring power of second chances and the timeless magic of romance. For in each other's arms, they had found solace, joy, and the promise of a love.

# 61. Beyond the Garden Gates

In the picturesque town of Rockford, nestled in the heart of New England's rolling hills, two souls found themselves ensnared in the delicate dance of love and societal expectations: Alice and Henry.

Alice, a widowed woman with a gentle spirit and a love for nature's beauty, tended to her sprawling garden with care, finding solace in the quiet tranquility of her surroundings. Henry, a ruggedly handsome gardener with a heart as tender as the flowers he nurtured, captured Alice's attention from the moment they met, his presence awakening long-dormant desires within her.

Their paths crossed one crisp autumn morning when Henry was hired to tend to Alice's garden, his green thumb and easy charm quickly endearing him to her heart. Drawn together by a shared love of nature and a desire for companionship, they found themselves embarking on a journey of friendship and discovery, their hearts entwined like the vines that climbed the garden walls.

As the seasons changed and the beauty of the garden bloomed anew, Alice and Henry found themselves falling deeper and deeper in love, their bond growing stronger with each passing day. But their happiness was short-lived as the whispers of society's disapproval began to spread, casting a shadow over their budding romance.

With judgmental eyes and wagging tongues threatening to tear them apart, Alice and Henry found themselves faced with an impossible choice: to bow to the pressures of convention and sacrifice their love, or to defy expectations and follow their hearts wherever they may lead.

In a moment of courageous defiance, Alice and Henry chose love over fear, stepping beyond the garden gates and into a world of uncertainty and possibility. With the beauty of the natural world as their witness and the strength of their love as their guide, they embarked on a journey of self-discovery and liberation, their hearts soaring as they embraced the freedom to love openly and unapologetically.

And as they walked hand in hand beneath the starry skies of Rockford, their laughter mingling with the rustle of leaves and the chirping of crickets, Alice and Henry knew that they had found their own little slice of heaven on earth. For in each other's arms, they had discovered the true meaning of love, acceptance, and the courage to live life on their own terms.

## 62. Crescent City Serenade

In the vibrant streets of 1950s New Orleans, where the sound of jazz filled the air and the scent of gumbo wafted from every corner, two souls found themselves entangled in a tale of temptation, redemption, and the seductive allure of the Crescent City: Marie and Johnny.

Marie, a sultry nightclub singer with a voice as smooth as bourbon and a spirit as fiery as the Louisiana sun, held court at the Blue Rising Club, captivating audiences with her siren song and mesmerizing presence. Johnny, a brooding young man with dreams of escape and a talent for trouble, found himself drawn to Marie's magnetic charm, his heart yearning for a taste of the freedom she embodied.

Their paths crossed one moonlit night when Johnny stumbled upon the Blue Rising Club, his curiosity piqued by the sultry strains of Marie's voice drifting out into the street. Drawn together by a shared love of music and a desire for something more, they found themselves swept up in a whirlwind of passion and danger, their hearts racing with the rhythm of the city.

As they danced through the dimly lit streets of the French Quarter, Marie and Johnny found themselves ensnared in a web of secrets and lies, their forbidden romance threatening to ignite a powder keg of emotions that could destroy them both. With danger lurking around every corner and temptation calling their names, they were forced to confront the demons of their pasts and the realities of their present in order to find their way back to each other.

In a moment of desperate reckoning, Marie and Johnny found themselves standing at a crossroads, their hearts laid bare and their souls exposed to the unforgiving gaze of the city that had shaped them. With the strains of jazz as their witness and the scent of magnolias in the air, they embraced the truth of their love and the promise of a future filled with endless possibility.

Marie and Johnny knew that they had found their own little slice of paradise in each other's arms. For in the heart of the Crescent City, they had discovered the true meaning of love, redemption, and the unbreakable bonds that could withstand even the darkest of nights.

## 63. Island Serenade

In the tropical paradise of 1960s Hawaii, where the ocean stretched out like a sapphire blanket and the palm trees swayed in the gentle breeze, two souls found themselves swept away by the rhythms of the island and the intoxicating magic of love: Lani and Kai.

Lani, a spirited island beauty with eyes as deep as the ocean and a smile as bright as the sun, spent her days tending to the lush gardens that surrounded her family's beachside resort, her heart overflowing with the warmth of aloha. Kai, a handsome young surfer with a carefree spirit and a love for adventure, roamed the waves of the Pacific with a sense of freedom that matched the endless horizon.

Their paths crossed one balmy afternoon when Kai stumbled upon Lani's family's resort, drawn by the promise of crystal-clear waters and white sandy beaches. Drawn together by a shared love of the ocean and a deep connection to the land, they found themselves embarking on a journey of discovery and romance, their hearts intertwined like the leis they exchanged.

As they explored the hidden treasures of the island and danced beneath the stars on moonlit beaches, Lani and Kai found themselves falling deeper and deeper in love, their bond growing stronger with each passing day. But their idyllic paradise was soon threatened by the pressures of tradition and the expectations of their families, who stood in the way of their happiness.

With the weight of their responsibilities bearing down on them and the specter of separation looming on the horizon, Lani and Kai were forced to confront the truth of their feelings and the depth of their love for each other. In a moment of reckless abandon, they threw caution to the wind and followed their hearts, embarking on a daring adventure that would test the limits of their courage and the strength of their commitment.

In the shadow of the majestic mountains and the whispers of the trade winds, Lani and Kai exchanged vows of love and devotion, their hearts soaring as they pledged themselves to each other for all eternity. With the melody of island music as their soundtrack and the scent of tropical flowers in the air, they danced together in celebration of their newfound freedom and the promise of a future filled with endless possibility.

Lani and Kai knew that they had found their own little slice of heaven in each other's arms. For in the heart of paradise, they had discovered the true meaning of love, loyalty, and the unbreakable bonds that could withstand even the strongest of storms.

## 64. The Delight of Togetherness

In the elegant streets of 1960s San Francisco, where the Golden Gate Bridge spanned the bay and the city skyline glittered in the sunlight, two souls found themselves drawn together by the simple pleasures of companionship and the joy of shared moments: Pamela and James.

Pamela, a refined socialite with a heart as warm as her smile and a passion for life's finer things, lived a life of luxury in her sprawling mansion overlooking the city, her days filled with charity galas and society events. James, a charming free spirit with a mischievous twinkle in his eye and a penchant for adventure, returned to San Francisco after years of globe-trotting, his presence injecting a breath of fresh air into Pamela's carefully curated world.

Their paths crossed one sunny afternoon when James unexpectedly showed up on Pamela's doorstep, his easy charm and infectious enthusiasm captivating her from the moment they reunited. Drawn together by the memories of their shared past and the promise of new adventures ahead, they found themselves embarking on a journey of rediscovery and reconnection, their hearts intertwining like the branches of a majestic oak tree.

As they roamed the streets of San Francisco, exploring hidden treasures and reliving old memories, Pamela and

James found themselves swept up in a whirlwind of laughter and love, their bond growing stronger with each passing day. But their newfound happiness was soon threatened by the demands of Pamela's social obligations and the expectations of those around them, who couldn't understand the depth of their connection.

With the weight of the world pressing down on them and the specter of loneliness lurking in the shadows, Pamela and James were forced to confront the truth of their feelings and the depth of their love for each other.

In the glow of the city lights and the warmth of each other's embrace, Pamela and James found solace in the beauty of the present moment and the promise of a future filled with endless possibility. With the skyline as their backdrop and the stars as their witnesses, they held each other in celebration of their love and the happiness they had found in each other's arms.

Pamela and James knew that they had found their own little slice of paradise in each other's company.

# 65. Whispers in the Moonlight

In the sun-kissed shores of 1950s French Riviera, where the azure waters lapped against the rugged cliffs and the scent of jasmine hung heavy in the air, two souls found themselves entangled in a web of mystery, allure, and forbidden passion: Lisa and Adrian.

Lisa, a captivating socialite with a flair for adventure and a secret past shrouded in mystery, moved through the glamorous world of high society with ease, her beauty and charm masking the truth of her troubled past. Adrian, a notorious thief with a heart of gold and a reputation for evading capture, found himself drawn to Lisa's enigmatic allure, his desire for redemption matched only by his longing for her embrace.

Their paths crossed one moonlit night when Lisa caught Adrian in the act of stealing jewels from a lavish gala, her curiosity piqued by his audacity and her heart stirred by his dangerous charm. Drawn together by a shared sense of intrigue and a desire for something more, they found themselves embarking on a dangerous game of cat and mouse, their hearts racing with the thrill of the chase and the promise of forbidden romance.

As they danced through the shadows of the French Riviera, eluding the authorities and unraveling the mysteries of Lisa's past, Adrian and Lisa found themselves ensnared in a dangerous game of deception and desire. With danger lurking around every corner and betrayal threatening to tear them apart, they were forced to confront the truth of their feelings and the risks they were willing to take for love.

In a moment of reckless abandon, Lisa and Adrian threw caution to the wind and surrendered to the undeniable pull of their passion, their hearts entwined like the vines that climbed the ancient cliffs above them. And as they stood together on the precipice of danger and desire, they knew that their love was worth any risk, any sacrifice, for in each other's arms, they had found solace, salvation, and the promise of a future filled with endless possibility.

As they disappeared into the night, their laughter mingling with the whispers of the sea and the rustle of the palm trees, Lisa and Adrian knew that their journey was far from over. For in the shadows of intrigue, they had discovered the true meaning of love, loyalty, and the irresistible allure of a life lived on the edge.

## 66. Sands of Destiny

In the ancient lands of Egypt, where the mighty Nile flowed like a lifeline through the desert sands and the echoes of history whispered through the corridors of power, two souls found themselves swept up in the tumultuous currents of ambition, betrayal, and undying love: Cleo and Marcus.

Cleo, a captivating queen with a heart as fierce as her ambition and a spirit as untamed as the desert wind, ruled over Egypt with grace and cunning, her beauty and intellect commanding the adoration of all who beheld her. Marcus, a valiant general with a loyalty as unwavering as his sword and a determination as unyielding as the pyramids themselves, pledged his allegiance to Rome, his destiny intertwined with the fate of an empire.

Their paths crossed one fateful day when Marcus arrived in Egypt, his legions marching triumphantly through the streets of Alexandria as Cleo looked on from her throne, her eyes ablaze with curiosity and desire. Drawn together by the irresistible pull of power and the promise of a new alliance, they found themselves embarking on a journey of political intrigue and forbidden passion, their hearts entwined like the serpent of the Nile.

As they navigated the treacherous waters of ancient politics and the shifting sands of destiny, Cleo and Marcus found themselves tested in ways they never imagined. With betrayal lurking in the shadows and enemies closing in on all sides, they were forced to confront the truth of their feelings and the sacrifices they were willing to make for love and power.

In a moment of desperate defiance, Cleo and Marcus defied the expectations of their empires and embraced their forbidden love, their hearts united against the chaos of war and the machinations of fate. And as they stood together amidst the ruins of fallen kingdoms and the whispers of history, they knew that their love was a force as powerful as the gods themselves, a beacon of hope in a world consumed by darkness.

As they rode into battle side by side, their love shining like a guiding star in the night sky, Cleo and Marcus knew that they were destined for greatness. For in the sands of destiny, they had found each other, and together, they thought they could conquer the world.

## 67. Racing Hearts

In the sun-drenched racetracks of 1960s California, where the roar of engines filled the air and the thrill of speed ignited passions, two souls found themselves caught in the whirlwind of love, rivalry, and fast-paced excitement: Elizabeth and Paul.

Elizabeth, a spirited race car driver with nerves of steel and a determination to conquer the track, lived life in the fast lane, her fiery spirit matched only by her love for the adrenaline rush of competition. Paul, a charming mechanic with a knack for fixing cars and a heart as free as the wind, found himself drawn to the world of racing, his desire to prove himself matched only by his longing for Elizabeth's affection.

Their paths crossed one fateful day when Elizabeth's car broke down on the racetrack, leaving her stranded and frustrated as Paul came to her rescue, his easy smile and quick wit instantly winning her over. Drawn together by a shared love of speed and a mutual desire for victory, they found themselves embarking on a journey of passion and rivalry, their hearts racing with the thrill of the chase and the promise of victory.

As they tore up the racetrack, battling against each other and the other drivers vying for glory, Elizabeth and Paul found themselves caught in a whirlwind of emotions and desires, their bond growing stronger with every turn of the wheel. But their heated competition was soon threatened by the specter of jealousy and the pressures of the racing world, threatening to tear them apart on and off the track.

With the stakes higher than ever and their hearts on the line, Elizabeth and Paul were forced to confront the truth of their feelings and the sacrifices they were willing to make for love. They threw caution to the wind and surrendered to the undeniable pull of their passion, their love burning brighter than the California sun.

Elizabeth and Paul knew that they had found their own little slice of paradise in each other's arms. For in the thrill of the chase and the heat of the competition, they had discovered the true meaning of love, loyalty, and the unbreakable bond that would carry them through all the twists and turns of life's racecourse.

## 68. A Cradle of Love

In the heartwarming neighborhoods of 1950s suburban America, where the scent of freshly cut grass wafted through the air and the laughter of children filled the streets, two souls found themselves embarking on the greatest adventure of all: parenthood. Meet Penny and David.

Penny, a kind-hearted homemaker with a smile that could light up a room and a nurturing spirit that knew no bounds, dreamed of starting a family and filling her home with the pitter-patter of little feet. David, a hardworking businessman with a heart as big as his ambitions and a love for Penny that knew no end, yearned to be a father and build a future with the woman he adored.

Their journey to parenthood took an unexpected turn one fateful day when a surprise bundle arrived on their doorstep, nestled snugly in a basket with a note that read: "Handle with love." Drawn together by the overwhelming sense of responsibility and the shared desire to provide a loving home, Penny and David embraced their newfound roles as parents, their hearts overflowing with joy and gratitude.

As they navigated the ups and downs of parenthood, from sleepless nights to endless diaper changes, Penny and David found themselves falling more deeply in love with each other and with the precious gift they had been given. With each coo and giggle, each milestone reached and each tender moment shared, they discovered the true meaning of family and the boundless capacity of the human heart to love.

In the cozy nursery they had lovingly prepared, surrounded by the soft glow of moonlight and the gentle hum of a lullaby, Penny and David rocked their bundle of joy to sleep, their hearts bursting with love and wonder at the miracle of life. And as they watched their little one drift off into dreams, they knew that their lives would never be the same again, forever enriched by the love of their precious bundle of joy.

As the years passed and their family grew, Penny and David looked back on those early days with fondness and gratitude, cherishing the memories they had created and the love that had blossomed in their hearts. For in the cradle of love they had built together, they had found the truest, most precious gift of all: the gift of family, and the gift of unconditional love.

## 69. Melodies of Joy

In the vibrant streets of 1950s Hollywood, where the stars shone brightly and the magic of the silver screen captivated audiences around the world, two souls found themselves swept up in the enchanting rhythm of love and laughter: Grace and Michael.

Grace, a talented actress with a heart as pure as her voice and a passion for performing that knew no bounds, graced the stages of Tinseltown with her beauty and charm, her every movement a dance, her every word a song. Michael, a dashing choreographer with a smile as bright as the sun and a talent for turning dreams into reality, brought the magic of dance to life on the big screen, his every step a symphony, his every gesture a masterpiece.

Their paths crossed one fateful day on the set of a Hollywood musical, where Grace found herself cast as the leading lady and Michael as the choreographer tasked with bringing her performance to life. Drawn together by their shared love of music and dance, they embarked on a journey of creativity and collaboration, their hearts beating in perfect harmony with the melodies of joy that filled the air.

As they danced through the streets of Hollywood, twirling and spinning in perfect rhythm, Grace and Michael found themselves falling in love amidst the magic of the silver screen. With each song they sang and each step they took, their bond grew stronger, their love deeper, until they could no longer deny the truth of their feelings.

In a moment of pure bliss, Grace and Michael surrendered to the music of their hearts, their love shining like a beacon in the night sky, illuminating the path to their shared destiny. And as they danced in each other's arms, their laughter ringing out like bells in the wind, they knew that they had found true happiness in each other's embrace.

As the final curtain fell and the credits rolled, Grace and Michael stood hand in hand, their hearts overflowing with love and gratitude for the journey they had taken together. For in the melodies of joy that filled their lives, they had found the truest, most precious gift of all: the gift of love, and the promise of a lifetime filled with music, laughter, and endless love.

## 70. Love's Cozy Retreat

In the quaint suburbs of 1950s America, where the aroma of freshly baked apple pie filled the air and the laughter of children echoed in the streets, two hearts found refuge in the warmth of their shared love: Margaret and Tony.

Margaret, a nurturing homemaker with a smile that could brighten the darkest of days and a knack for turning a house into a home, dreamed of building a cozy nest where love would flourish and memories would be made. Tony, a hardworking man with a heart as vast as his dreams and a devotion to Margaret that knew no bounds, yearned to provide for his beloved and create a sanctuary where their love could thrive.

Their journey to creating their love nest began one crisp autumn day when they stumbled upon a charming cottage nestled in a picturesque corner of the suburbs, its inviting facade and lush garden beckoning them closer. Drawn together by their shared vision of a life filled with love and laughter, Margaret and Tony seized the opportunity to turn the cottage into their own little haven, a retreat from the hustle and bustle of the outside world.

As they settled into their new home, Margaret and Tony discovered the joy of building a life together, one filled with simple pleasures, shared dreams, and unwavering devotion. With each passing day, their bond grew stronger, their connection deeper, as they faced life's challenges with courage and grace, knowing that they had each other to lean on.

In their cozy retreat, surrounded by the warmth of their love and the comfort of familiar routines, Margaret and Tony found solace and contentment in each other's arms, cherishing the moments they shared and the dreams they dared to dream. And as they looked out at the world from the windows of their cottage, they knew that they had found their own little slice of paradise, a haven of love and happiness where their hearts would always find refuge.

## 71. Western Trails of Love

In the vast expanse of the American frontier in the 19th century, where the rugged landscapes stretched as far as the eye could see and the promise of a new life beckoned to those with courage and determination, two souls found themselves swept up in the epic saga of love, adventure, and destiny: Sarah and William.

Sarah, a spirited pioneer with a heart as wild as the untamed wilderness and a spirit as free as the wind, set out on a journey westward in search of freedom and opportunity, her eyes ablaze with the promise of adventure. William, a rugged explorer with a sense of duty as strong as his resolve and a longing for a place to call home, ventured into the unknown with dreams of carving out a life for himself and his loved ones.

Their paths crossed on the dusty trails of the Oregon Trail, where Sarah's wagon train crossed paths with William's scouting party, their destinies intertwined by the call of the frontier and the promise of a new beginning. Drawn together by the challenges and dangers of the untamed wilderness, they embarked on a journey of discovery and perseverance, their hearts beating in unison with the rhythm of the land.

As they traversed the rugged terrain of the American West, facing untold hardships and forging bonds of friendship and camaraderie along the way, Sarah and William found themselves falling in love amidst the beauty and majesty of the frontier. With each sunrise and sunset, each obstacle overcome and each triumph achieved, their love grew stronger, their connection deeper, as they embraced the untamed spirit of the land and the untamed desires of their hearts.

But their journey perilous, as they encountered hostile natives, treacherous landscapes, and the ever-present threat of danger lurking in the shadows. With the odds stacked against them and their futures uncertain, Sarah and William were forced to confront the true cost of their love and the sacrifices they were willing to make for the chance to build a life together on the untamed frontier.

They realized that the true measure of their love lay not in the destination, but in the journey itself, in the trials and tribulations they had faced together and the bonds of love and loyalty that had sustained them through it all. And as they stood together atop a windswept hill, gazing out at the vast expanse of the American West stretching out before them, they knew that they had found their own little piece of heaven on earth, a place where their love could flourish and their spirits could soar forevermore.

# 72. Love Amidst the Storm of War

In the tumultuous backdrop of World War I, where the echoes of gunfire pierced the air and the specter of death loomed over the battlefield, two souls found solace and sanctuary in each other's arms: Catherine and Edward.

Catherine, a compassionate nurse with a heart as resilient as her spirit and a devotion to healing that knew no bounds, tended to the wounded soldiers with unwavering courage and compassion, her every action guided by the desire to ease their pain and suffering. Edward, a courageous young soldier with a sense of duty as strong as his love for Catherine, found himself drawn to her kindness and strength, his heart yearning for the warmth of her embrace amidst the chaos of war.

They met in the dimly lit confines of a field hospital, where Catherine tended to Edward's wounds with gentle hands and soothing words, her presence a beacon of hope amidst the darkness of war. Drawn together by the shared horrors of battle and the fragile beauty of life, they found comfort and solace in each other's company, their hearts intertwining amidst the chaos and uncertainty of the world around them.

As they navigated the trials and tribulations of war, from the frontlines of battle to the quiet moments of respite in the hospital wards, Catherine and Edward found themselves falling deeply in love amidst the turmoil and tragedy of the world. With each passing day, their bond grew stronger, their connection deeper, as they clung to each other with a fierceness born of desperation and desire.

With the horror of war haunting their every move, Catherine and Edward were forced to confront the fragility of life and the sacrifices they were willing to make for the chance to be together.

They realized that their love was worth fighting for, worth risking everything for, even in the face of insurmountable odds. And as they stood together amidst the chaos and destruction of war, their hearts united in love and defiance, they knew that they had found in each other a kindred spirit, a soulmate, and a love that would endure even amidst the darkest of storms.

They knew that, come what may, their love would remain as eternal and unyielding as the stars that shone overhead, a beacon of hope amidst the chaos and destruction of war.

## 73. Hearts on the Road

In the vibrant world of 1960s America, where the open road stretched out before them like an endless promise and the roar of engines filled the air with excitement, two souls found themselves drawn together by the thrill of adventure and the call of the highway: Rose and Johnny.

Rose, a spirited young woman with a love for freedom as boundless as the horizon and a spirit as wild as the wind, craved the excitement of life on the road, her every step guided by the rhythm of the journey and the promise of new beginnings. Johnny, a charming roustabout with a guitar slung over his shoulder and a twinkle in his eye, lived for the thrill of the open road, his heart beating in time with the hum of the engine and the roar of the crowd.

Their paths crossed at a roadside diner, where Rose caught Johnny's eye with her fierce independence and adventurous spirit, her presence a beacon of light amidst the darkness of his nomadic existence. Drawn together by the allure of the highway and the promise of freedom, they embarked on a journey of self-discovery and adventure, their hearts racing with the thrill of the open road and the excitement of the unknown.

As they traveled from town to town, their hearts intertwined amidst the roar of the engine and the rush of the wind, Rose and Johnny found themselves falling deeply in love amidst the ever-changing landscape of America. With each passing mile, their bond grew stronger, their connection deeper, as they embraced the freedom of the open road and the joy of being together.

Along the way they faced run-ins with the law to clashes with rival road crews, but they didn't let it deter them. They surrendered to the undeniable pull of their passion, their love burning bright amidst the chaos and excitement of life on the road.

Rose and Johnny knew that they had found in each other a kindred spirit, a soulmate, and a love that would endure even amidst the twists and turns of the open road.

# 74. Love in the Rally

In the bustling town of Jefferson's Landing in 1950s America, where the sense of community ran deep and the bonds of friendship were unbreakable, two souls found themselves caught up in the whirlwind of small-town life and unexpected romance: Alice and Jack.

"Attention, everyone! I have an important announcement to make," Alice declared, standing at the front of the town hall, her voice ringing out with determination.

The crowd quieted down, turning their attention to Alice as she spoke passionately about the need to preserve the town's natural beauty and protect it from the encroachment of industrial development.

"We can't let them destroy what makes Jefferson's Landing so special," Alice continued, her eyes shining with conviction. "We need to rally together and fight for our community!"

As the townsfolk murmured in agreement, Jack couldn't help but admire Alice's fiery spirit and unwavering dedication to their town. Stepping forward, he found himself drawn to her, his heart pounding with a newfound sense of admiration and attraction.

"I couldn't agree more, Alice," Jack chimed in, his voice strong and sure. "We need to stand together and protect what's ours."

Alice turned to him, a spark of recognition igniting in her eyes. "Jack, I didn't realize you felt the same way," she said, a hint of surprise in her voice.

Jack smiled, feeling a surge of warmth at her words. "I've always admired your passion and commitment to this town, Alice. I'd be honored to stand by your side and fight for what's right."

And in that moment, amidst the cheers of their fellow townsfolk, Alice and Jack knew that they had found in each other not only kindred spirits, but also the beginnings of a love that would endure even amidst the challenges and triumphs of small-town life.

## 75. Sparkling Dreams

In the glitzy world of 1950s glamour and allure, where the lights of Broadway dazzled and the allure of luxury beckoned, two women found themselves swept up in a whirlwind of desire and adventure: Marilyn and Doris.

Marilyn, a vivacious blonde bombshell with a smile that could light up Times Square and a thirst for the finer things in life, captivated audiences with her charm and charisma, her every move a spectacle of elegance and grace. Doris, her sharp-witted brunette companion with a heart as bold as her ambition and a knack for getting what she wanted, stood by Marilyn's side as they navigated the glitz and glamour of New York City's high society.

Their escapades took them from the bright lights of Broadway to the opulent ballrooms of Manhattan's elite, where Marilyn dazzled audiences with her performances and Doris charmed the city's most eligible bachelors with her wit and charm. But amidst the whirl of parties and paparazzi, Marilyn and Doris found themselves drawn to the allure of something more than fame and fortune: love.

As they danced the night away and basked in the adoration of their admirers, Marilyn and Doris found themselves falling for two charming gentlemen who captured their hearts in unexpected ways. Marilyn, drawn to the dashing billionaire with a penchant for extravagance and a heart of gold, found herself swept off her feet by his lavish gifts and declarations of love. Doris, on the other hand, found herself drawn to the ruggedly handsome journalist with a keen intellect and a passion for adventure, his every word a tantalizing glimpse into a world beyond the glitz and glamour of the city.

But as they embarked on whirlwind romances filled with passion and excitement, Marilyn and Doris soon realized that love was far more complicated than they ever imagined. With their hearts torn between desire and duty, they were forced to confront the true nature of their feelings and the sacrifices they were willing to make for the chance at true happiness.

Marilyn and Doris finally realized that true love was not about diamonds and designer gowns, but about finding someone who accepted them for who they truly were, flaws and all. And as they embraced the simple pleasures of companionship and understanding, they knew that they had found in each other the truest, most precious gift of all: a friend who would stand by their side through thick and thin, no matter where their adventures took them.

## 76. Secrets Beneath the Surface

In the sunny coastal town of Santa Catalina in the swinging 1960s, where the ocean breeze carried the scent of salt and adventure, two souls found themselves entangled in a web of mystery and romance: Jennifer and David.

"Welcome aboard the Glass Bottom Boat, folks! I'm Jennifer, your tour guide for today," Jennifer greeted with a bright smile as the passengers boarded the boat.

David, a charming aerospace engineer with a penchant for secrecy and a heart full of hidden desires, observed Jennifer from a distance, his curiosity piqued by her adventurous spirit.

"Mind if I tag along?" David asked, approaching Jennifer with a charming smile.

Jennifer glanced at him, intrigued by his sudden appearance. "Sure, but just remember to keep your hands and feet inside the boat at all times," she replied with a playful wink.

As they set off on their underwater expedition, Jennifer guided the group through the crystal-clear waters, pointing out colorful fish and exotic coral reefs along the way. David listened intently, captivated by Jennifer's passion for the ocean and her knowledge of its mysteries.

"You seem to know a lot about this place," David remarked, watching Jennifer with admiration.

"I've always been fascinated by the ocean. There's so much we have yet to discover down there," Jennifer replied, her eyes sparkling with excitement.

Their conversation flowed effortlessly as they explored the underwater world together, their shared love for adventure forging a bond between them that neither could deny.

But as they delved deeper into the mysteries of the ocean floor, David sensed that Jennifer was hiding something, a secret lurking beneath the surface that threatened to tear them apart.

"Jennifer, there's something I need to tell you," David began, his voice tinged with uncertainty.

Before he could say another word, Jennifer silenced him with a finger to his lips, her eyes locking with his in a silent plea for understanding.

"I know, David. And I have secrets of my own," Jennifer confessed, her voice barely above a whisper.

In that moment, as they stood together amidst the beauty and wonder of the underwater world, Jennifer and David realized that their love was worth fighting for, worth risking everything for, even if it meant diving headfirst into the unknown.

And as they embraced the mysteries of the ocean and the secrets of their hearts, Jennifer and David knew that they had found in each other a kindred spirit, a partner in adventure, and a love that would endure even amidst the storms of life.

## 77. Paths Unraveled

In the lush jungles of the Dutch East Indies in the 1960s, where the air was thick with humidity and the sounds of exotic wildlife filled the air, two souls found themselves on a journey of self-discovery and redemption: Sarah and Daniel.

Sarah, a determined young doctor with a passion for healing and a heart full of compassion, traveled to the remote village of Selampang to serve the local community, her every step guided by a sense of duty and a desire to make a difference. Daniel, a troubled surgeon with a haunted past and a longing for redemption, arrived in Selampang seeking refuge from his demons, his every move shrouded in mystery and intrigue.

Their paths crossed one fateful day when Sarah stumbled upon Daniel performing surgery in a makeshift clinic, his hands steady and his focus unwavering despite the chaos around him. Drawn together by their shared commitment to healing and their desire to make a difference, they embarked on a journey of self-discovery and redemption, their hearts intertwined amidst the lush jungles and hidden dangers of the Dutch East Indies.

As they worked side by side to treat the villagers and confront the challenges of life in the jungle, Sarah and Daniel found themselves drawn to each. With each patient they healed and each obstacle they overcame, their bond grew stronger, their connection deeper, as they explored the depths of their souls and the true meaning of redemption.

They realized that their love was worth fighting for, worth risking everything for, even if it meant facing their darkest fears and confronting the unknown. And as they stood together amidst the lush jungles of the Dutch East Indies, their hearts united in love and determination, they knew that they had found in each other a kindred spirit, a partner in healing, and a love that would endure even amidst the twists and turns of the spiral road ahead.

## 78. Fairground Serendipity

In the bustling excitement of the 1962 World's Fair in Seattle, where the air was electric with the promise of innovation and discovery, two souls found themselves swept up in a whirlwind of chance and destiny: Samantha and Michael.

Samantha, a free-spirited young woman with dreams as vast as the fairgrounds themselves and a sense of wonder that knew no bounds, wandered through the exhibits with awe and excitement, her every step a testament to her adventurous spirit and thirst for new experiences. Michael, a charming pilot with a heart as free as the skies and a passion for adventure, found himself drawn to Samantha's infectious enthusiasm and zest for life, his every move guided by a sense of curiosity and a longing for connection.

Their paths crossed at the fairgrounds, where Samantha stumbled upon Michael performing daredevil stunts in his vintage biplane, his every maneuver a breathtaking display of skill and daring. Drawn together by the thrill of the fair and the excitement of the moment, they embarked on a journey of discovery and adventure, their hearts racing with the promise of the unknown.

As they explored the wonders of the fair together, from the Space Needle to the futuristic exhibits showcasing the latest in technology and innovation, Samantha and Michael found themselves falling for each other amidst the excitement and wonder of it all. With each attraction they visited and each moment they shared, their bond grew stronger, their connection deeper, as they discovered the true magic of the fair: the chance to find love in the most unexpected of places.

With the fair drawing to a close and the real world looming on the horizon, Samantha and Michael discovered the true nature of their feelings and the sacrifices they were willing to make for the chance at true happiness.

They realized that their love was worth fighting for, worth risking everything for, even if it meant saying goodbye to the excitement of the fair and the thrill of the moment. And as they stood together amidst the fading lights of the fairgrounds, their hearts united in love and determination, they knew that they had found in each other a kindred spirit, a partner in adventure, and a love that would endure even amidst the challenges and triumphs of life beyond the fairgrounds.

## 79. Roman Discovery

In the romantic streets of 1950s Rome, where the air was filled with the scent of blooming flowers and the promise of adventure, two souls found themselves on a journey of self-discovery and unexpected love: Amelia and Giovanni.

As the sun cast its golden rays over the ancient city, Amelia, disguised as an ordinary tourist, wandered through the bustling streets, her heart yearning for escape from the confines of her royal duties.

"Excuse me, miss, are you lost?" Giovanni's voice broke through Amelia's thoughts, his warm gaze meeting hers with genuine concern.

Amelia hesitated for a moment, caught off guard by Giovanni's sudden appearance. "No, I'm just... exploring," she replied, her voice tinged with uncertainty.

Giovanni smiled, his eyes twinkling with mischief. "Well, you've certainly picked the right city for it. Allow me to be your guide," he offered, extending his hand with a charming grin.

Amelia hesitated, her heart racing with excitement at the prospect of adventure. "I... I suppose I could use a guide," she admitted, taking Giovanni's hand with a shy smile.

Together, they roamed the cobblestone streets and ancient ruins of Rome, their laughter filling the air.

"You know, you're not like any other tourist I've ever met," Giovanni remarked, his gaze lingering on Amelia with a hint of curiosity.

Amelia chuckled, a blush creeping into her cheeks. "I suppose that's because I'm not really a tourist," she confessed, her eyes sparkling with mischief.

Giovanni's expression softened, a smile playing at the corners of his lips. "I thought as much. There's something about you... something special," he admitted, his voice low and sincere.

As the day drew to a close and the sun began to set over the city, Amelia and Giovanni found themselves standing on a quiet rooftop, the twinkling lights of Rome spread out before them in all its glory.

"I never expected today to turn out like this," Amelia confessed, her heart overflowing with gratitude for the unexpected adventure and the newfound connection she shared with Giovanni.

Giovanni turned to her, his eyes sparkling with emotion. "Neither did I. But I'm glad it did," he whispered, leaning in closer until their lips met in a tender kiss, sealing their love amidst the timeless beauty of Rome.

## 80. Mischief in Millbrook

In the quaint town of Millbrook in 1960s America, where the streets buzzed with the energy of small-town life and the promise of mischief lurked around every corner, two souls found themselves entangled in a series of comical mishaps and unexpected romance: Lucy and Max.

Lucy, a spirited young woman with a penchant for trouble and a heart as big as her dreams, worked at the local diner, her every day filled with laughter and excitement as she navigated the ups and downs of small-town living. Max, a charming young mechanic with a mischievous twinkle in his eye and a knack for getting into trouble, found himself drawn to Lucy's infectious energy and irrepressible spirit, his every move a testament to his determination to win her heart.

Their paths crossed one fateful day when Lucy's car broke down on the side of the road, leaving her stranded in the middle of nowhere with no way to get to work. Max, passing by on his way to the auto repair shop, stopped to offer his assistance, his charming smile and easygoing nature instantly putting Lucy at ease.

As they worked together to fix Lucy's car, they found themselves embroiled in a series of comical mishaps and misadventures, from grease stains to runaway tools, their laughter filling the air as they bonded over their shared love of mischief and mayhem.

"I swear, trouble seems to follow you wherever you go," Max remarked, wiping grease off his hands with a grin.

Lucy laughed, a sparkle in her eye. "And yet, here you are, right in the middle of it all," she teased, nudging him playfully.

Their banter continued as they worked side by side, their hearts growing closer with each passing moment as they discovered a shared love for life's little adventures.

And as they embraced the unpredictable twists and turns of life in Millbrook, Lucy and Max knew that they had found in each other a kindred spirit, a partner in mischief, and a love that would endure even the most troublesome of encounters.

## 81. Stars Aligned

In the glitz and glamour of 1960s Hollywood, where the bright lights of fame and fortune shone down upon the city of dreams, two souls found themselves caught in the whirlwind of showbiz and unexpected romance: Ava and Marcus.

Ava, a talented young actress with a heart full of ambition and a fire that burned brighter than the Hollywood sign itself, graced the silver screen with her undeniable presence and captivating performances. Marcus, a charismatic yet enigmatic musician with a passion for music and a longing for connection, found himself drawn to Ava's magnetic charm and irresistible allure, his every move a testament to his desire to win her heart.

They met when Marcus, rehearsing for his latest Broadway production, stumbled upon Ava's audition for the lead role in the same play. Drawn together by their shared love for the stage and the spotlight, they embarked on a journey of discovery and passion, their hearts entwined amidst the glitz and glamour of showbiz.

As they rehearsed their lines and honed their performances together, Ava and Marcus found themselves falling for each other amidst the hustle and bustle of Hollywood's bright lights and bustling streets. With each scene they acted out and each note they sang, their bond grew stronger, their connection deeper, as they explored the depths of their souls and the true meaning of love.

But their romance faced challenges, as they navigated the complexities of fame and fortune amidst the pressures of showbiz and the scrutiny of the public eye. With their hearts on the line and their dreams hanging in the balance, they realized that their love was worth fighting for.

As they stood together amidst the glittering lights of Hollywood, their hearts united in love and determination, they knew that they had found in each other a kindred spirit, a partner in passion, and a love that would endure even amidst the challenges and triumphs of life in the spotlight.

## 82. Fields of Sunlight

In the rolling hills of 1970s Tuscany, where the golden fields of sunflowers stretched as far as the eye could see, two souls found themselves entwined in a tale of love and longing amidst the beauty of the Italian countryside: Isabella and Matteo.

Isabella, a spirited young woman with a heart as free as the wind and a spirit as radiant as the Tuscan sun, tended to the sunflower fields with care and devotion, her every step guided by a love for the land and a longing for connection. Matteo, a rugged yet gentle farmer with a soul as deep as the earth and a love for the simple pleasures of life, found himself drawn to Isabella's magnetic charm and irresistible passion, his every move a testament to his desire to win her heart.

Their paths crossed when Matteo, wandering through the sunflower fields, stumbled upon Isabella as she tended to the crops. Drawn together by their shared love for the land and the beauty of nature, they embarked on a journey of discovery and romance amidst the golden fields of Tuscany.

As they worked side by side to nurture the sunflower fields and harvest the bountiful crops, Isabella and Matteo found themselves falling deeper in love amidst the breathtaking beauty of the Italian countryside. With each sunrise they witnessed and each sunset they shared, their bond grew stronger, their connection deeper, as they explored the depths of their hearts and the true meaning of love.

As they stood together amidst the golden fields of sunflowers, their hearts united in love and determination, they knew that they had found in each other a kindred spirit, a partner in passion, and a love that would endure even amidst the challenges and triumphs of life in the Tuscan countryside.

## 83. Tango of Temptation

In the smoky depths of 1940s Buenos Aires, where the sultry strains of tango filled the air and secrets lingered in the shadows, two souls found themselves entangled in a web of desire and deception amidst the seductive allure of the Argentine nightlife: Elena and Alejandro.

Elena, a mysterious and alluring woman with a past shrouded in mystery and a heart hardened by betrayal, danced her way through the dimly lit clubs of Buenos Aires, her every move a tantalizing invitation to temptation. Alejandro, a dashing yet enigmatic casino owner with a thirst for danger and a hunger for power, found himself drawn to Elena's magnetic charm and irresistible allure, his every move a testament to his desire to possess her.

Their paths crossed at the infamous Club Gilda, where Elena captivated the audience with her mesmerizing dance moves and smoldering gaze. Alejandro, entranced by her beauty and captivated by her grace, offered her a job as the star attraction at his casino, his every word laced with promises of wealth and luxury.

As they danced the forbidden dance of desire and temptation, Elena and Alejandro found themselves entangled in a dangerous game of seduction and betrayal, their hearts racing with the thrill of the chase and the promise of passion.

"You dance like no one else I've ever seen," Alejandro remarked, his voice husky with desire as he watched Elena move across the dance floor.

Elena smiled, her eyes flashing with mischief. "And you know just how to make a girl feel special," she purred, her voice dripping with seduction.

With each tango they danced and each secret they shared, their bond grew stronger, their connection deeper, as they explored the depths of their desires and the true meaning of love.

"I can't promise you a life without danger, but I can promise you my love," Alejandro whispered, his voice filled with sincerity as he held Elena close.

Elena sighed, her heart aching with longing. "And I can promise you my loyalty, no matter what may come," she vowed, her eyes locked with his in a silent pledge of devotion.

They knew that they had found in each other a kindred spirit, a partner in passion, and a love that would endure even amidst the dangers and temptations of life in Buenos Aires.

## 84. Sails of Destiny

In the vast expanse of the Pacific Ocean, where the salty breeze carried tales of adventure and the horizon held the promise of uncharted lands, two souls found themselves caught in the tumultuous waves of destiny and desire: Isabella and Captain Diego.

Isabella, a spirited and independent woman with a yearning for adventure that matched the vastness of the sea itself, roamed the bustling port of San Francisco, her every step echoing with the determination to defy the expectations of society and chart her own course. Captain Diego, a rugged and seasoned sailor with a heart as vast as the ocean and eyes that mirrored the depths of the sea, found himself drawn to Isabella's fiery spirit and unwavering resolve, his every move guided by the call of the open sea and the promise of distant shores.

They me when Isabella, seeking passage to the distant shores of Alaska in search of adventure and fortune, found herself aboard Captain Diego's majestic ship, the pride of the Pacific. Bound together by the shared allure of the unknown and the promise of new beginnings, they set sail into the endless blue, their hearts filled with anticipation and their spirits alive with the thrill of the voyage.

As they navigated the treacherous waters of the Pacific, Isabella and Captain Diego found themselves drawn to each other amidst the vastness of the sea and the timeless beauty of the stars above. With each passing day, their bond grew stronger, their connection deeper.

For love they would brave the storms of the sea and the trials of the unknown. As they stood together beneath the starlit sky, their hearts united in love and determination, they knew that they had found in each other a kindred spirit, a partner in adventure, and a love that would endure even amidst the vastness of the Pacific and the trials of the open sea.

## 85. Trail of Honor

In the rugged wilderness of the American Southwest, where the sun scorched the earth and the winds whispered tales of bravery and betrayal, two souls found themselves entangled in a tale of redemption and romance amidst the untamed beauty of the desert: Maria and Juan.

Maria, a fierce and resilient woman with a heart as wild as the desert itself and a spirit unbroken by the hardships of life, roamed the vast expanse of the Arizona desert, her every step echoing with the determination to seek justice for those who had wronged her. Juan, a rugged and honorable cowboy with a past shrouded in mystery and a heart as steadfast as the mountains, found himself drawn to Maria's fiery spirit and unwavering resolve, his every move guided by a sense of duty and a longing for redemption.

Maria was tracking down a band of outlaws who had stolen her family's land, when she found herself in need of assistance in the unforgiving desert. Juan, riding across the arid landscape in search of his own redemption, stumbled upon Maria's camp, his heart stirred by the sight of her fiery determination and unwavering resolve.

Bound together by a shared sense of honor and a desire to right the wrongs of the past, Maria and Juan set out on a journey of justice and redemption, their hearts united in a common cause amidst the harsh beauty of the desert.

"You're one tough woman, Maria," Juan remarked, his voice gruff yet filled with admiration as they rode side by side.

Maria smiled, a glint of mischief in her eyes. "Tough times call for tough measures, Juan," she replied, her tone soft yet determined.

With each passing day, their bond grew stronger, their connection deeper.

They faced off against ruthless outlaws and treacherous terrain in their pursuit of truth and honor.

"We're in this together, Maria," Juan declared, his voice unwavering as they stood face to face with danger.

Maria nodded, her gaze steady and determined. "Together till the end, Juan," she vowed, her heart filled with courage and resolve.

In a moment of clarity, they realized that their love was worth fighting for, worth risking everything for, even if it meant braving the dangers of the desert and the trials of the open trail. And as they stood together beneath the blazing sun, their hearts united in love and determination, they knew that they had found in each other a kindred spirit, a partner in justice, and a love that would endure even amidst the harsh beauty of the American Southwest and the trials of the open trail.

# 86. Tropics of Love

In the lush paradise of 1960s Hawaii, where the scent of plumeria filled the air and the gentle waves of the Pacific Ocean lapped against the shores, two souls found themselves swept away in a melody of love and adventure amidst the tropical splendor: Serena and Keoni.

Serena, a vibrant and free-spirited young woman with a love for music as boundless as the ocean itself, lived her days immersed in the rhythm of the islands, her every step guided by the sway of the palm trees and the whispers of the trade winds. Keoni, a charming and adventurous pilot with a heart as vast as the sky and a love for the thrill of flight, found himself drawn to Serena's infectious laughter and the beauty of her soul, his every move a testament to his desire to capture her heart.

Their paths crossed one enchanting day when Serena, performing at a beachside luau beneath the starlit sky, captured Keoni's attention with her mesmerizing voice and graceful dance. Entranced by her beauty and captivated by her spirit, Keoni found himself drawn to Serena like a moth to a flame, his heart soaring on the wings of love amidst the tropical paradise of Hawaii.

As they explored the hidden treasures of the islands and danced beneath the moonlit sky, Serena and Keoni found themselves falling deeper in love amidst the tropical splendor of Hawaii.

"You dance as though the waves themselves are guiding your steps," Keoni remarked, his voice soft as he watched Serena twirl gracefully under the moonlight.

Serena smiled, her eyes sparkling with joy. "In Hawaii, the ocean speaks to everyone who listens," she replied, her voice filled with the magic of the islands.

With each passing day, their bond grew stronger, their connection deeper, as they shared tales of island legends and dreams of a future filled with love and laughter.

"Sometimes, the currents of life can be unpredictable," Keoni mused, his brow furrowed with concern as they watched the sunset over the horizon.

Serena nodded, her hand reaching out to grasp his. "But as long as we're together, we can weather any storm," she declared, her voice filled with unwavering determination.

They realized that their love was worth fighting for, even if it meant braving the storms of the sea and the trials of life on the islands. And as they stood together beneath the swaying palms, their hearts united in love and determination, they knew that they had found in each other a kindred spirit, a partner in adventure, and a love that would endure even amidst the paradise of Hawaii.

## 87. Skies of Destiny

In the expansive skies over the Korean Peninsula, where the roar of jet engines drowned out the cries of war and the clouds offered fleeting sanctuary, two souls found themselves intertwined in a tale of courage and camaraderie amidst the perilous missions of the U.S. Navy: Linda and Paul.

Linda, a steadfast and resilient nurse with a heart as tender as it was brave, tended to the wounded with unwavering dedication, her every action a testament to her compassion and strength. Paul, a daring and skilled pilot with a spirit as untamed as the wind and a heart as noble as it was daring, soared through the heavens with fearless determination, his every maneuver a dance with destiny amidst the chaos of war.

They first met on the deck of the USS Saratoga, where Linda tended to the injured and Paul prepared for another perilous mission over enemy territory. Drawn together by the shared dangers of war and the fleeting moments of peace, they forged a bond amidst the chaos of conflict, their hearts united in a common cause amidst the uncertainty of the battlefield.

As Paul flew his missions and Linda tended to the wounded, they found solace in each other's company amidst the turmoil of war. With each passing day, their bond grew stronger, their connection deeper, as they shared tales of bravery and sacrifice, and dreams of a future free from the horrors of war.

They faced the dangers of combat and the uncertainties of life on the front lines. With their hearts on the line and the skies filled with danger, Linda and Paul were forced to confront the true nature of their feelings and the sacrifices they were willing to make for the chance at true happiness.

As they stood together on the deck of the USS Saratoga, their hearts united in love and determination, they knew that they had found in each other a partner in courage, and a love that would endure even amidst the perils of war and the uncertainty of the skies.

## 88. Sands of Time

In the bustling streets of 1960s Cairo, where the scent of spices hung heavy in the air and the mysteries of the desert whispered secrets of the past, two souls found themselves entangled in a tale of adventure and romance amidst the ancient wonders of Egypt: Sally and Ahmed.

Sally, a spirited and adventurous archaeologist with a passion for uncovering the mysteries of the past, roamed the labyrinthine alleyways of Cairo, her every step guided by the allure of ancient artifacts and the promise of discovery. Ahmed, a dashing and enigmatic guide with a deep connection to the desert and a heart as vast as the endless sands, found himself drawn to Sally's adventurous spirit and insatiable curiosity, his every move a testament to his desire to protect her from the dangers that lurked in the shadows.

Sally was on a quest to uncover the lost treasures of the Pharaohs, found herself in need of a guide to navigate the treacherous sands of the desert. Ahmed, drawn to Sally's determination and passion for adventure, offered his services as her guide, his heart stirred by the possibility of uncovering the secrets of the ancient world together.

Bound together by a shared love for history and the promise of adventure, Sally and Ahmed found their hearts intertwined amidst the ancient wonders of Egypt.

As they explored the hidden tombs and temples of the desert, Sally and Ahmed found themselves drawn to each other amidst the timeless beauty of the ancient world.

"This place is filled with stories waiting to be told," Sally remarked, her eyes sparkling with excitement as they ventured deeper into the desert.

Ahmed nodded, a smile playing on his lips. "And I am grateful to share this adventure with you, Sally," he replied, his voice warm with sincerity.

With each passing day, their bond grew stronger, their connection deeper, as they shared tales of ancient civilizations and dreams of unlocking the secrets of the past.

But there were those who sought to keep the secrets of the past buried.

"We must tread carefully, Sally. There are those who would stop at nothing to protect what lies hidden in these sands," Ahmed cautioned, his gaze scanning the horizon for signs of danger.

Sally nodded, her determination unwavering. "I will not let fear stand in the way of uncovering the truth, Ahmed. Together, we can overcome any obstacle."

Their hearts were united in love and determination, and they knew that they had found in each other a partner in adventure, and a love that would endure even amidst the sands of time.

## 89. Ocean Serenade

In the bustling port town of Harbor Haven, where the salty breeze kissed the cheeks of sailors and the sea whispered tales of adventure, lived a spirited young woman named Anna. She longed for the thrill of the open sea, her heart yearning for adventure beyond the confines of her small coastal town.

One fateful day, as Anna stood gazing out at the endless expanse of the ocean, a dashing sailor named James caught her eye. With his rugged charm and piercing blue eyes, he swept her off her feet, his laughter echoing like the call of a siren in the wind.

Their romance blossomed against the backdrop of the high seas, as James whisked Anna away on a journey filled with excitement and intrigue. They sailed to distant shores, exploring hidden coves and dancing beneath the stars on moonlit decks.

As they sailed into uncharted waters, they faced fierce storms and treacherous seas, their love tested by the elements that threatened to tear them apart.

Together, they braved the perils of the ocean, their love guiding them like a beacon of light in the darkness.

And so, as they sailed into the sunset, hand in hand, Anna and James knew that their love was as boundless as the ocean itself. For in the vast expanse of the sea, they had found a love that would endure for all eternity.

## 90. Whispered Secrets

In the bustling city of Riverdale, where the neon lights flickered and the streets buzzed with excitement, lived a young woman named Lucy. She spent her days working as a secretary in a crowded office, her nights filled with dreams of love and romance.

One evening, as Lucy sat alone in her apartment, a handsome stranger moved in next door. His name was Jack, and he was charming and witty, with a smile that could light up the darkest of nights. From the moment they met, there was an undeniable spark between them, like a flame waiting to be ignited.

As the days turned into nights, Lucy and Jack found themselves drawn to each other like magnets. They would often meet in the hallway, their conversations flowing effortlessly as they shared stories and laughter late into the night.

One night, as they leaned against the railing of the staircase, Jack turned to Lucy with a mischievous glint in his eye. "You know, Lucy," he said, his voice low and husky, "I think Mrs. Jenkins is starting to suspect something."

Lucy chuckled, brushing a stray lock of hair behind her ear. "She's always been a busybody," she replied. "But I don't care what she thinks. As long as we're together, that's all that matters."

Their laughter echoed through the empty hallway, mingling with the soft hum of the city outside. In that moment, Lucy felt a warmth spread through her chest, a feeling of contentment she had never known before.

Mrs. Jenkins, watched their every move with a critical eye, determined to uncover their whispered secrets. And Jack's ex-girlfriend, Sylvia, lurked in the shadows, plotting to win him back at any cost.

Yet, despite the challenges they faced, Lucy and Jack refused to let anything come between them. They would steal moments together whenever they could, sharing secrets and dreams in the soft glow of the moonlight.

As their love deepened, Lucy and Jack found solace in each other's arms, their whispered confessions binding them together in ways they never thought possible. And when Jack finally confessed his love for Lucy, she knew that her dreams had finally come true.

In the bustling city of Riverdale, where the neon lights flickered and the streets buzzed with excitement, two hearts found refuge in the quiet moments shared between whispered secrets.

## 91. Farewell to Paris

In the enchanting streets of Paris, where the aroma of freshly baked croissants lingered in the air and the Seine River whispered tales of romance, lived a young woman named Adele. She was a dreamer, her heart filled with wanderlust and a longing for adventure.

Adele's life took a turn when she met a captivating young artist named Henri. With his passionate soul and artistic flair, he swept her off her feet, whisking her away on a whirlwind romance through the cobblestone streets of Paris.

Their love blossomed like the vibrant blooms in the Jardin des Tuileries, each moment filled with laughter and shared dreams. They danced beneath the starlit sky, their footsteps echoing through the city streets as they lost themselves in the magic of Parisian nights.

But as the seasons changed and the winds of war swept across the land, Adele's world was turned upside down. Henri was called to serve his country, leaving Adele behind with nothing but memories of their time together.

The last time Adele saw Paris, it was ablaze with the colors of autumn, the leaves falling like tears from the sky. She stood on the banks of the Seine, watching as the city she loved faded into the distance, a bittersweet reminder of the love she had lost.

As the years passed and the world changed around her, Adele clung to the memories of her time in Paris, holding onto the hope that one day, she would be reunited with Henri once more.

## 92. Whispers of the Heartland

In the expansive vistas of the American South, where golden fields stretched as far as the eye could see and the wind carried the faint scent of wildflowers, lived a young woman named Sarah. She was a dreamer, her spirit as boundless as the endless prairies that surrounded her.

Sarah's world was forever changed when she met a charismatic young man named John. With his warm smile and gentle manner, he ignited a spark within her that felt like the sun breaking through the clouds.

Their love blossomed amidst the rolling plains and endless skies of the Raintree County, as Sarah and John lost themselves in the beauty of the land and the depth of their feelings.

"Sarah, do you see that?" John whispered, pointing to the horizon where the sun dipped below the fields in a blaze of orange and gold. "That's how you make me feel, like every moment with you is a sunset that never fades."

Sarah smiled, her eyes sparkling with affection. "John, you have a way with words," she said softly, leaning into his embrace. "But it's not just the sunsets. It's the way you make me feel alive, like I'm truly free."

As tensions rose and the Civil War loomed on the horizon, Sarah and John found themselves torn apart by forces beyond their control.

Separated by war and circumstance, Sarah and John embarked on separate journeys, each haunted by the memories of their lost love.

In the end, it was their enduring love for each other that brought them back together, as they rediscovered the beauty of the home and the strength of their hearts amidst the trials of war.

Sarah and John found solace in the whispers of their hearts, their love as timeless and enduring as the land itself.

## 93. Courageous Hearts

In the rugged hills of Spain, where the echoes of history reverberated through ancient castles and sun-kissed vineyards, lived a spirited young woman named Elena. She was a beacon of strength and resilience, her fiery spirit matched only by the passion that burned in her heart.

Elena's world was forever changed when she crossed paths with a daring guerrilla fighter named Diego. With his unwavering courage and magnetic presence, he ignited a flame within her that blazed brighter than the Spanish sun.

Their love story unfolded amidst the turmoil of war, as Elena and Diego joined forces to fight against the tyranny of an oppressive regime. Together, they braved the dangers of battle and the uncertainty of the future, their hearts bound by a shared sense of purpose and unwavering determination.

As they stood side by side on the battlefield, Elena turned to Diego with a fierce determination in her eyes. "We will fight until the very end," she declared, her voice ringing with conviction. "For our freedom, for our people, for our love."

Diego nodded, his gaze steady and unwavering. "Together, we are unstoppable," he replied, his hand reaching out to grasp hers in a silent pledge of solidarity.

They faced impossible odds and insurmountable obstacles at every turn. Yet, through it all, Elena and Diego remained resolute in their commitment to each other and to their cause.

In the end, it was their courageous hearts that carried them through the darkest of times and brought them to the dawn of a new era. As they stood victorious against the forces of oppression, Elena, Diego and their love were a beacon of light in a world shrouded in darkness.

## 94. Love's Rhythms

In the enchanting streets of Buenos Aires, where the rhythms of tango filled the night and the scent of jasmine lingered in the air, lived a young woman named Isabella. She was a vision of grace and beauty, her laughter like music to the ears of all who heard it.

Isabella's world was forever changed when she crossed paths with a charming musician named Alejandro. With his smooth melodies and charismatic charm, he swept her off her feet, igniting a passion within her that she had never known before.

Their romance blossomed amidst the sultry nights and vibrant energy of Buenos Aires, as Isabella and Alejandro danced beneath the starlit sky, their hearts beating in time to the rhythm of their love.

As they strolled along the cobblestone streets, Alejandro turned to Isabella with a smile. "You are the melody to my song," he whispered, his eyes filled with adoration.

Isabella blushed, her heart fluttering at his words. "And you are the music to my dance," she replied, her voice soft with emotion.

Their unwavering devotion to each other that carried them through the trials and tribulations, emerging stronger and more deeply in love than ever before.

Isabella and Alejandro's love story became a timeless serenade.

# 95. Whispered Secrets

In the elegant corridors of London's high society, where whispers of scandal and intrigue danced on the lips of the elite, lived a sophisticated woman named Victoria. She was a captivating presence, her wit and charm drawing admirers from all corners of the city.

Victoria met Edward, a charming diplomat with a smile as disarming as it was enchanting. From the moment their eyes met across a crowded ballroom, a spark ignited between them, setting off a chain of events neither could have predicted.

Their romance unfolded amidst the backdrop of glittering ballrooms and lavish soirées, as Victoria and Edward danced through the night, their hearts entwined in a whirlwind of desire and longing.

As they strolled through Hyde Park, Edward turned to Victoria with a smile. "You are the most enchanting woman I have ever met," he whispered, his eyes filled with adoration.

Victoria blushed, her heart fluttering at his words. "And you, my dear Edward, are a gentleman of unparalleled charm," she replied, her voice soft with affection.

As they navigated the intricacies of Victorian society, Victoria and Edward found themselves entangled in a web of secrets and lies that threatened to tear them apart.

Their unwavering commitment to each other that brought them back together, stronger and more deeply in love than ever before.

Victoria and Edward's love story became a delicate dance of deception, a testament to the power of love to overcome even the greatest of obstacles and endure.

## 96. Jailhouse Blues

In the gritty streets of Memphis, where the blues wailed and the rhythm of life pulsed like a heartbeat, lived a young man named Johnny. He was a rebel with a guitar, his soul ablaze with the fire of rock 'n' roll.

Johnny's life took an unexpected turn when he found himself behind bars, his dreams shattered and his future uncertain. But it was within the confines of the jailhouse that he discovered a new rhythm, a beat that resonated deep within his soul.

With each strum of his guitar and each note he sang, Johnny found solace in the music, his voice echoing through the halls.

As he performed for his fellow inmates, Johnny caught the attention of a music producer named Lisa. With her sharp wit and keen eye for talent, she saw in Johnny a star waiting to be born.

Their collaboration sparked a revolution, as Johnny's raw talent and untamed energy captivated audiences far and wide. From smoky bars to packed arenas, he electrified the stage with his presence, his music igniting a fire in the hearts of all who listened.

But fame came with its own set of challenges, as Johnny found himself grappling with the pressures of stardom and the temptations of the industry. And when his past came back to haunt him, he was forced to confront the demons he thought he had left behind.

In the end, it was the power of music that saved Johnny, as he rediscovered his passion and purpose in the midst of chaos. With each chord he strummed and each lyric he sang, he found redemption in the heartbeat rhythm of blues and rock 'n' roll.

In the gritty streets of Memphis, where the blues wailed and the rhythm of life pulsed like a heartbeat, Johnny's journey from jailhouse rebel to rock 'n' roll legend was complete.

## 97. Echoes of the Emerald Isle

In the quiet village of Glenwood, nestled among the rolling hills of Ireland, lived a young man named Liam. After years of city life in America, he felt a pull back to his roots, to the land of his ancestors.

Liam's heart stirred as he stepped off the train, greeted by the familiar sights and sounds of home. The air was crisp with the scent of wildflowers, and the gentle melody of the nearby stream soothed his soul.

As he walked through the village square, Liam caught sight of a spirited young woman named Nora. Her fiery red hair danced in the breeze, and her eyes sparkled with mischief as she went about her day.

Their paths crossed again and again, each encounter leaving Liam more captivated by Nora's charm and beauty. He found himself drawn to her laughter, to the way she moved with grace and confidence through the village streets.

In the evenings, Liam would sit by the hearth in the local pub, listening to tales of love and adventure as he sipped on a pint of ale. And always, his thoughts would drift back to Nora, the girl who had stolen his heart with a single glance.

One day, as they walked along the winding paths of the countryside, Liam mustered the courage to confess his feelings to Nora. "I've never felt more at home than I do when I'm with you," he admitted, his voice trembling with emotion.

Nora smiled, her eyes shining with affection. "And I've never met anyone quite like you, Liam," she replied softly, reaching out to take his hand in hers.

Their love blossomed like the wildflowers that dotted the landscape, growing stronger with each passing day. They shared stolen moments beneath the shade of ancient oak trees, their laughter mingling with the rustle of leaves in the breeze.

As they stood together, hand in hand, beneath the starlit sky, they knew that their love was destined to endure, echoing through the ages like the song of the Emerald Isle.

## 98. Oil and Romance

In the sprawling oil fields of Texas, where fortunes were made and lost with the turn of a drill, lived a rugged independent oil driller named Jake. He was a man of the land, his hands calloused from years of hard work and his heart as untamed as the wild Texas plains.

Jake's life changed forever when he crossed paths with a sophisticated society woman named Emily. With her refined manners and elegant charm, she was like a breath of fresh air amidst the dusty oil fields.

Their worlds collided amidst the backdrop of business and intrigue, as Jake and Emily found themselves drawn to each other against all odds. Despite their differences in background and upbringing, they couldn't deny the undeniable spark that ignited between them.

As they worked together to navigate the complexities of the oil industry, Jake and Emily found themselves entangled in a web of deceit and betrayal. But amidst the chaos and uncertainty, their love blossomed like a wildflower in the desert, resilient and untamed.

In the heart of Texas, where the oil flowed like liquid gold and the sun beat down upon the land, Jake and Emily's romance burned bright against the backdrop of the oil fields. And as they stood together, hand in hand, they knew that their love was as enduring as the Texas sky, stretching out endlessly before them.

# 99. Starlit Stars

In the vibrant streets of Los Angeles, where aspirations shimmered like city lights against the evening sky, lived a young actress named Mia. She had ventured to the City of Angels with dreams of gracing the silver screen, her spirit ablaze with ambition and hope.

Mia's life took an unexpected turn when she crossed paths with a talented jazz musician named Luke. With his soulful melodies and effortless charm, he struck a chord within her, igniting a spark of passion that illuminated her heart like a shooting star.

Their romance bloomed amidst the glitz and glamour of the city, as Mia and Luke pursued their dreams with unwavering determination. They wandered the streets of Los Angeles together, lost in the rhythm of their footsteps and the promise of a brighter future.

As they performed in intimate venues and auditioned for roles, Mia and Luke found solace in their shared love for music and the arts. They encouraged each other to persevere, to chase their dreams with unwavering dedication even in the face of adversity.

One evening, as they stood beneath the starlit sky, Mia turned to Luke with a smile. "This moment feels like magic," she whispered, her eyes alight with wonder.

Luke took her hand in his, his heart overflowing with affection. "With you by my side, every moment feels like a symphony," he replied, his voice filled with sincerity. "Together, we can conquer the world."

But they faced setbacks and disappointments along the way, their dreams sometimes seeming just out of reach.

Yet, through it all, Mia and Luke remained steadfast in their love for each other, their bond growing stronger with each passing day. And as they stood on the cusp of success, ready to conquer the city that had once seemed so daunting, they knew that their love was the brightest star in their constellation.

# 100. Saved by Seattle

In the bustling city of Seattle, where the rain kissed the streets and the Space Needle pierced the sky, lived a widowed father named Jack. He had devoted himself to raising his young son, Sam, after the loss of his beloved wife, their hearts still healing from the ache of her absence.

Jack's life took an unexpected turn when Sam called into a late-night radio show, pouring out his heart about missing his mother and wishing for a new wife for his dad. Their heartfelt conversation captured the attention of listeners far and wide, including a woman named Sarah who listened from across the country.

As fate would have it, Sarah found herself drawn to Jack's story, her heart stirred by the sincerity and love in his son's words. Despite living thousands of miles away in Baltimore, she couldn't shake the feeling that she was meant to be a part of their lives.

Their paths converged amidst the backdrop of love and longing, as Jack and Sam embarked on a journey of healing and discovery. With the help of Sam's matchmaking efforts and a little bit of serendipity, they found themselves on a cross-country adventure to meet Sarah, the woman who had captured their hearts from afar.

In the end, it was their shared journey of love and loss that brought them together, their hearts finding solace in the warmth of each other's embrace. And as they looked out over the city skyline, bathed in the soft glow of the moonlight, they knew that their love was written in the stars.

## 101. Duty and Devotion

In the sun-drenched streets of a seaside town, where the ocean breeze whispered secrets of love and adventure, lived a young man named Nathan. He was a dreamer with a heart of gold, his spirit yearning for something more than the life laid out before him.

Nathan's life changed when he enlisted in the Navy, determined to find purpose and honor amidst the turmoil of war. As he navigated the challenges of boot camp, he crossed paths with a nurse named Paula, a spirited young woman whose laughter was like music to his ears.

Their connection blossomed amidst breaks during the rigors of training.

"Hey, Nathan, catch!" Paula tossed a ball to him during a picnic ball game.

Nathan caught it with a grin. "Thanks, Paula. You always know how to brighten up the day."

Paula chuckled. "Just trying to keep the morale up. We're in this together, right?"

Nathan nodded, feeling a warmth spread through his chest. "Absolutely. We'll get through this together."

As they navigated the complexities of military life, Nathan and Paula found themselves tested in ways they never could have imagined.

"This long-distance thing is tough, Paula," Nathan confessed one evening over a crackling phone line. "But I promise, I'm coming back to you."

Paula's voice was filled with determination. "I believe in you, Nathan. Stay safe out there."

Yet, through it all, their love remained steadfast and true, a beacon of hope amidst the chaos of war.

In the end, it was their love that carried them through the darkest of times, their hearts united against the backdrop of a world at war.

"I love you, Nathan," Paula whispered as they embraced on the dock, his ship preparing to set sail once more.

Nathan held her close, the scent of her hair mingling with the salt in the air. "I love you too, Paula. I'll be back before you know it."

And as he sailed off into the horizon, Nathan knew that their love would endure, and the power of the human spirit was able to overcome even the greatest of obstacles.

# Other Books from Seniorality

To find your next book visit:

**www.amazon.com/author/seniorality**

Where you will find:

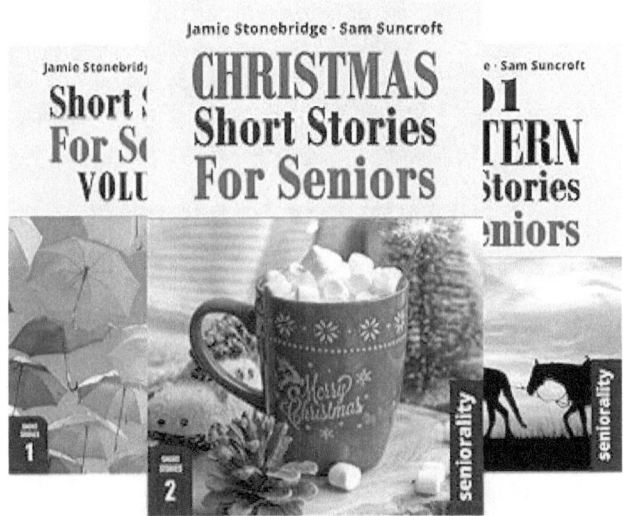

**Short Stories**

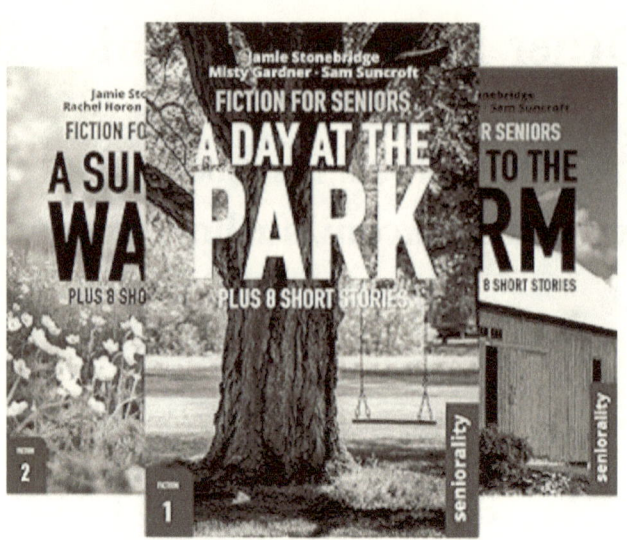

**Fiction for Seniors**

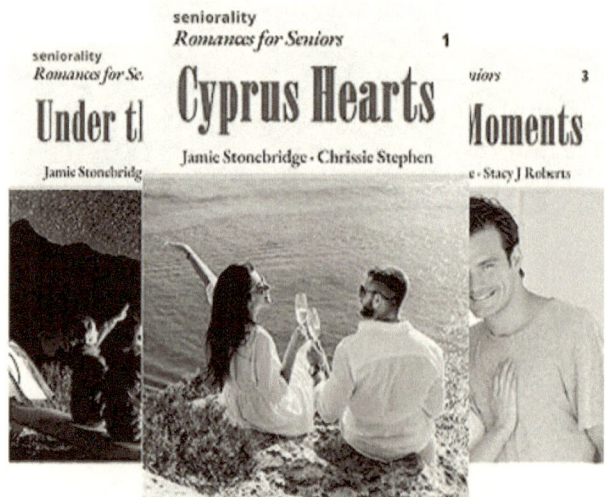

**Romances for Seniors**

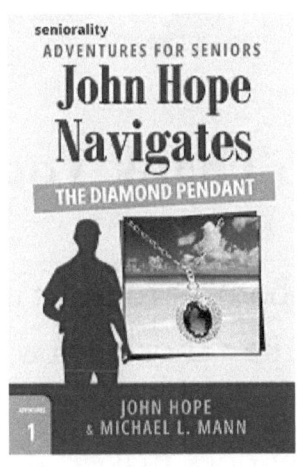

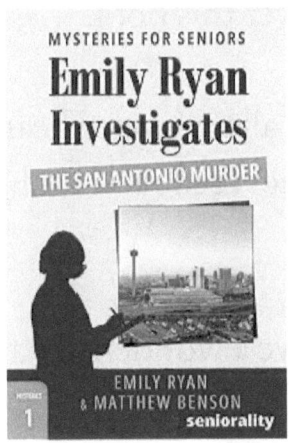

Find these books and many more
by searching on Amazon for
**'seniorality'**
or visit:

**www.amazon.com/author/seniorality**

# Thank You

If you enjoyed this book or found it useful, we'd be very grateful if you'd write a short review on Amazon.

Your support really does make a difference and helps other people discover this book.

We personally read all reviews to hear how the books are being used, to collect feedback, and get ideas for future stories.

Thank you and have a wonderful day!

www.ingramcontent.com/pod-product-compliance
Lightning Source LLC
Chambersburg PA
CBHW020638220526
45464CB00001B/198